THE
DIET
WHISPERER

12-Week Reset Plan

Dr Paul Barrington Chell &
Dr Monique Hope-Ross

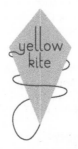

yellow
kite

First published in Great Britain in 2022 by Yellow Kite
An imprint of Hodder & Stoughton
An Hachette UK company

3

The information in this book is not intended to constitute medical advice, nor is it intended to replace or conflict with the advice given to you by your doctor or other health professional. Before embarking on the plans set out in this book, you should discuss them with your doctor, especially if you have any medical condition or if you are taking any medication. The author and publisher disclaim any liability directly or indirectly from the use of the material in this book by any person.

Author photo © Tamara Peel

A CIP catalogue record for this title is
available from the British Library

Trade Paperback ISBN 978 1 399 70185 3
eBook ISBN 978 1 399 70186 0

Typeset in Sabon LT by Palimpsest Book Production Ltd,
Falkirk, Stirlingshire

Printed and bound in Great Britain by Clays Ltd, Elcograf S.p.A.

Hodder & Stoughton policy is to use papers that are natural, renewable and recyclable products and made from wood grown in sustainable forests. The logging and manufacturing processes are expected to conform to the environmental regulations of the country of origin.

Yellow Kite
Hodder & Stoughton Ltd
Carmelite House
50 Victoria Embankment
London EC4Y 0DZ

www.yellowkitebooks.co.uk

'Thanks Dr Paul and Dr Monique, my husband lost
36 pounds in weight and is no longer diabetic.'
Nina, USA

'Thanks to all at Diet Whisperer HQ. You have changed
my life. I lost 80 pounds, and I am now the same weight
at 45 that I was in my teens. Life has completely changed
as my mental and physical health have blossomed.
God bless you all. Thank you soooooooo much.'
Sam, Australia

'This book should be in every hotel room and every school.
It is quite simply life-changing.'
John, Ireland

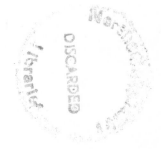

With eternal thanks to our mothers,
Maureen and Claire

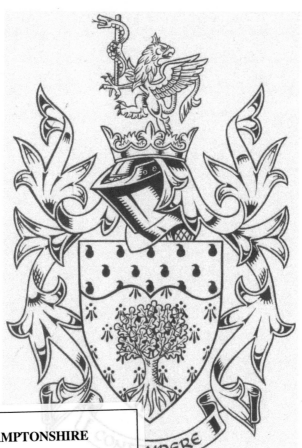

CONTENTS

ABOUT THE AUTHORS   ix

ABOUT THIS BOOK   xi

INTRODUCTION   1

PART ONE: THE ROAD TO OBESITY

1. THE OBESITY PANDEMIC   13

2. WHAT IS FOOD?   23

3. YOUR GUT MADE SIMPLE   29

4. CARBOHYDRATES   35

5. FATS   51

6. PROTEINS   63

7. GUT BUGS: YOUR FELLOW TRAVELLERS   69

8. GOOD FAT, BAD FAT   78

9. DIET MYTHS   90

10. FAT STORAGE HORMONES   96

PART TWO: THE ROAD FROM OBESITY

11. FAT ADAPTATION   111

12. THE ANCIENT PRACTICE OF FASTING   120

13. THE RHYTHM OF LIFE   129

PART THREE: THE WHISPERER PLANS

14. THE DIET WHISPERER SECRETS   147

15. YOUR PERSONAL GOALS   155

16. THE 12-WEEK RESET PLAN: FOOD   162

17. THE 12-WEEK RESET PLAN: WEEKS 1–4   171

18. THE 12-WEEK RESET PLAN: FASTING FITNESS   178

19. THE 12-WEEK RESET PLAN: WEEKS 5–8   183

20. THE 12-WEEK RESET PLAN: WEEKS 9–12   189

21. THE 12-WEEK RESET PLAN: WHAT NEXT?   197

22. THE 12-WEEK RESET PLAN: MEAL PLANS
AND RECIPES   200

GLOSSARY   252

NOTES   264

FURTHER READING   279

ACKNOWLEDGEMENTS   280

INDEX   281

ABOUT THE AUTHORS

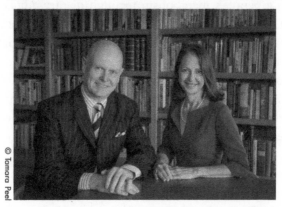

© Tamara Peel

Dr Paul Barrington Chell, MB ChB FRCOphth DO(RCSI)
Dr Monique Hope-Ross, MB ChB BAO FRCP FRCS FRCOphth DO

Paul and Monique are award-winning hospital doctors and researchers, with over 50 years of treating patients as consultant ophthalmic surgeons. At the pinnacle of their careers, they stepped aside to take on an exciting project. Instead of treating patients face-to-face in one place, they are now able to give help to people all over the world. Switching from treatment medicine to preventative medicine is proving to be their biggest and proudest achievement to date.

With new technology, books and the internet, it is possible to reach many more people. And rather than 'treating' the complications of obesity and metabolic disease, they can reach out and prevent those diseases in the first place.

Preventative medicine through nutrition and weight loss,
rather than pills, surgery and tears for the consequences.

Paul says: As doctors we knew we should be giving people hope for a healthy life through nutrition and prevention. We had to make that change, and we had to stand up as a voice for preventative medicine. Currently, medical prevention is effectively non-existent worldwide. And the medical community knows nothing about treating obesity, and nothing about nutrition. As doctors, too often we work in a system that rewards us for waiting for complications to appear, decades after the time when we should be intervening, helping and preventing future disease.

For decades we had seen the amazing results of reducing obesity, and correcting people's metabolism through dietary advice.

Today we have people in every corner of the world benefiting from the Diet Whisperer Plans. People whose lives have been totally transformed through nutrition. Untold numbers, now with reduced risks of heart disease, cancer or all of the dreadful complications of diabetes. This is the way forward for every person. For us the chance to reach millions worldwide, and give them happier, healthier and longer lives, is our greatest ambition yet.

We have now set up the Diet Whisperer Foundation, a charity funded by us, and through book sales, so we may reach out to the most vulnerable, weakest and youngest in society, and help them escape the 'obesity trap' and its terrible consequences. And to lobby government for intervention on nutrition, childhood obesity and corporate 'Big Food' harm.

Welcome to The Whisperer Family and thank you for reading the book. May we help your dreams come true.

Paul and Monique
Founders of The Diet Whisperer, www.diet-whisperer.com
and The Diet Whisperer Foundation

Paul and Monique have five university degrees, are diplomates of the Royal College of Surgeons of England and Ireland and are Fellows of four Royal Medical Colleges in the United Kingdom.

They have each delivered over 100 invited scientific lectures, have written many book chapters and have over 100 scientific publications, abstracts and communications to their names. They have both been scientific reviewers for international scientific journals. At home and abroad, they have lectured for over 20 years on nutrition, wellness and weight loss.

Paul and Monique have been presidents of five national and international learned medical societies. They have created the Diet Whisperer Foundation, a charity to help the most vulnerable, weakest and youngest in society to get help to escape the 'obesity trap'.

Outside of work they are both keen skiers. They started doing triathlons in their fifties. Paul did his first Olympic distance triathlon in 2016, at the age of 55, and Monique her first Ironman 140.6 in 2019 at the age of 59.

ABOUT THIS BOOK

Salad. I can't bear salad. It grows while you're eating it you know.

Alan Ayckbourn

A NEW LIFE, A NEW YOU

Firstly, a very big welcome to the Diet Whisperer. Monique and I wrote this book for all like-minded individuals: anyone wanting to lose weight *and* keep it off. And we'll certainly show you how to do that.

But it's about very much more than just your weight; it's about putting you in control and helping you improve your mental and physical health. This book is about empowering you to feel better, every day. Learn what makes you groggy, tired, mentally fogged up, and generally feeling lethargic and tired. Learn how to regain that spring in your step and feel alive, happy and on top of the world. You have a right to that, and right now. And we will show you how, in the clearest of ways.

FROM BOWEL DISEASE, THROUGH ARTHRITIS TO DIABETES AND HEART DISEASE

Find out exactly how food influences all human chronic inflammatory diseases, leaving people in pain and disabled for decades, with doctors treating symptoms with pills, rather than the cause with diet. Understand which foods make us ill, and how. When you've finished reading, you will be empowered for a new life, a new you, with you firmly back in control.

AVOIDING YO-YO DIETING

We know from science that diets work for a while, but eventually fail. Sound familiar?

The whisperer plan is not a fad diet. It is a journey, where you learn how *small changes* can make a massive difference to your weight and wellness, permanently. On the journey you will learn facts that will *shatter* long-held beliefs and preconceptions. The whole idea of the *whisperer reset plan* is to put you firmly back in control of your own body. You will choose your target weight, set your goals and achieve them. You will learn the foods that make you ill. You will see *immediate results* from your actions, as you join us on this exciting journey.

WHO IS THE BOOK DESIGNED FOR?

It is a book for men and women, young or old. While it is not a medical textbook, we hope doctors and medical students will enjoy it too, as nutrition is not on the medical radar. Doctors who have read it have told us it changed their personal and professional lives. We have pitched it at anyone who is inquisitive to know more about the relationship between food, illness and weight. Our readers share a common goal; they know that their current nutrition is causing them harm, illness and weight gain. Many tell us they have lost their sparkle. Their get-up-and-go. That fantastic appetite they had as kids. The ability to know exactly which foods are great and which are poisoning them. And they feel out of control and unable to get help.

The Diet Whisperer is a family where no one points fingers. Where we are all here to help, and where you will regain your zest for life.

IMPORTANT

PLEASE, PLEASE, please, continue with your current diet until you have read every word, in every chapter, in order. We know from our feedback that those who do this get the best results. By the time you get to the *reset plans* you'll fully understand them, and that is the time to change your diet. So, get stuck into your pizza and beer and enjoy them with your new read!

If you asked me which part of the book was the most important, of course I'd say all three! But I want to emphasise just how important the first section is. By reading it in order, you will build all the necessary knowledge and new terms will be explained; the whole story will emerge. You don't have to learn. The responsibility for your learning is with us, not you.

EUREKA MOMENTS: THE MOMENT THE PENNY DROPS

I can promise you, and I do mean *promise you*, you will find some eureka moments in every chapter. They often happen where you least expect them. We finish each chapter with a summary, *Chapter Whisperings*, and there is also a glossary at the back of the book.

You do not need any medical or scientific knowledge to read this book; just a desire to be leaner, healthier and to live longer. We understand that you are mad keen to lose 26 pounds (12 kg) in 12 weeks, or similar, but it is important you go steadily through this book, chapter by chapter, building your knowledge, for a completely different outlook on life. The new you. And importantly, it will put you in a position to help your loved ones too.

Monique has written the chapters on the microbiome, circadian rhythm and wellness, and Part Three, *The Whisperer Plans*. I'm afraid you'll have to put up with me for the rest. For the record, this has been a joint project for the last 20 years. Start to finish, we've loved every minute of the journey, helped so many people and worked tirelessly to make this project work for you. When you've regained complete, 100 per cent control over your own body's metabolism and weight, join us on the website and let us know how you're doing. Making you happy, fit and well makes us happy at Whisperer HQ 😊.

METABOLIC SYNDROME AND DIABETES

If you have type 2 diabetes and would like to give yourself a chance of reversing it, or if you have pre-diabetes, or metabolic syndrome, this book could be of the utmost, life-changing importance to you. Invest your time in learning about food, your fat, your fat storage hormones and how they interact. Don't worry about any of these terms for now, they will all become second nature by the end. You will need your doctor on board to adjust your medications, as you will lose weight rapidly. There is no single cure, pill or magic bullet. But, when you've finished the book, you will understand enough to free yourself from the control of the diet companies and the noxious food sellers. You will be in control of your own destiny. You will be able to choose your weight and, most importantly, control it long-term. On our website there are lots of resources to help improve your health. We encourage you to do the fun quiz before and after reading the book. It's confidential, but will show you how much your knowledge has changed. Just go to diet-whisperer.com/quiz.

And if you register you will receive our blogs and health bulletins on the latest science and medical issues of the day. It's time for you to become your own diet whisperer and take control over your nutrition, metabolism and weight. Learn to help yourself and your loved ones. That's the essence of what we're about: learning, then spreading the word; helping others and improving your karma.

Thanks for getting this far. We hope you enjoy the journey.

Welcome to the Diet Whisperer family.

Paul and Monique

To help us help others, please spread the word. Buy the books for friends and family. Every book sold means more money for the Whisperer Foundation, giving hope to the weakest, youngest and most vulnerable in our society and helping them free themselves from the 'obesity trap'. Links are available at www.diet-whisperer.com. Help us fight the fight.

INTRODUCTION

If I had an hour to save the world, I would spend the
first 55 minutes defining the problem and only five
minutes finding the solution.

Attributed to Albert Einstein

UNDERSTANDING THE PROBLEM

Einstein defines what is wrong with every commercial or fad diet
in the world. They concentrate on the solution. Dieters lose weight,
regain the weight, and pay again. Corporate diet companies are
con artists, with a perfect business model: *you fail and then you
pay again.*

The truth is, almost any form of calorie restriction will cause some
weight loss in the short term. In other words, all diets are bound to
work for a while, and then fail. Inevitably, consistently, and every
time. This is not a matter of opinion, but an irrefutable scientific
fact.[1] And the diet companies fleecing their flock are not stupid enough
to put themselves out of business by giving you a solution that actually works! They want and expect you to return.

The reasons for failure are not controversial. Firstly, diets will
inevitably fail if the dieter does not understand exactly *what* caused
the fat to arrive in the first place. It really is as simple as that. And
people think they do, but as you'll discover, they don't. Secondly,
most diets are horrible and unsustainable long-term. How long can
you survive on bowls of tasteless lettuce?! And neither should you.
Eating foods you don't like is not a requirement, as you'll learn.
And people do not understand that body fat is a sign of a broken
engine, just like a smoking exhaust on a car is a sign of an engine
problem. Our body's engine is called our metabolism; this is the
chemical processes by which we extract energy from our food, so we

may walk, see and think! When our metabolism (engine) goes awry, rather than a smoking exhaust it shows up as body fat.

When I was a keen third-year medical student, standing at the bedside in my first clinical attachment, my professor asked me, 'What is the diagnosis?'. The patient was yellow and unmistakably jaundiced. 'Jaundice, sir,' I answered, with some confidence. He let me know, unforgettably, that jaundice was a *sign* and not a *diagnosis*. And so it is with obesity! Obesity is a *sign* that our *metabolic engine* is suffering. This is called the temporal relationship: the order in which things occur. And it's the opposite way round to what I thought, and I'm willing to bet to what you thought too. In my medical school days, we were taught that obesity *caused* metabolic problems. We now know it is the other way round: metabolic problems cause obesity.[2]

Firstly, and crucially, we will teach you the mechanisms in your body that make you fat. And we will teach you exactly, why you get fat, and later how to shift it.

CONS VERSUS INCOMPETENCE

I'm certainly not a conspiracy person, and usually follow Hanlon's razor: 'Never attribute to malice that which can be explained by stupidity.' Nevertheless, realising you've been conned is a bitter pill to swallow. And you need to know what to avoid, and what to be wary of.

WE CAN HELP YOU

Healthcare professionals are among the worst people to advise you about diet and nutrition. Not because they don't care – I'm sure most do. But they were taught badly, believing that fat makes us fat, when the truth is that fat is our only hope to become thin. And no, saturated fat does not cause heart disease; the real culprit is processed foods, refined carbohydrates and sugar. More on this later.

When I visited hospitals as a child the overwhelming smell was of disinfectant; now it's toast! Over the years I have seen failure upon failure from people with good intentions, but without the knowledge to help you. My advice is to steer well clear of these well-intentioned people, put on the blinkers, and plough your own furrow. As you will learn, it's a real (nutritional) minefield out there.

Our governments, in some of the richest countries in the world, produce nutritional guidelines that are 40 years out of date; they tell us to eat mainly carbs, some protein and a little fat, which makes us fat and sick.

And as for diet companies, ask yourself *how* they continue to exist. Failure. Enough said.

JOIN MY GYM

Then there are the con men and women who tell you that exercise will make you lose weight; come join my gym! They make TV shows for ritual humiliation of their victims. And people watch this and believe it to be true. Let me state with absolute scientific certainty: EXERCISE WILL NOT MAKE YOU LOSE WEIGHT: FACT. Repeat as often as is necessary! Even people who exercise will tell you, 'Oh, that can't be right, I lost weight from running,' forgetting to tell you that they also radically changed their eating, which is the only way to lose weight. We expose all the dietary myths in Chapter 9. And before you misquote me, exercise in moderation is essential for both fitness and health. Just not for weight loss – as you'll learn.

BIG FOOD

Breakfast cereal companies, cake shops, fruit juice producers, chocolate bar sellers, fast-food sellers, muffin makers, the list is endless.

Let's be clear, these people do not sell food. They sell something that was once some form of food, but they converted it into junk that is bad for human beings. The processing of once good foods creates garbage, not food. An orange eaten is food. An orange juiced, yep you guessed it, *is garbage*. More on this poison later.

Corporate food scientists work tirelessly to produce the *'bliss point'* in their foods. They know the harm caused by added sweetness or additional fructose, but they will do anything to get you hooked and back for more. And human addictions to carbs and sugars are very, very strong. Fizzy drinks are just the same too. The diet versions are also highly addictive. You have been warned. Imagine the yachts in the marina with the food corporate moguls toasting the pharma magnates, clinking glasses, and saying, 'We're selling more food, so more people coming your way. Cheers.' It's as serious as the tobacco industry, which went on killing people for years after they knew the harm. The only difference is that with food harm, our governments are completely unwilling to act. This stance is unwise, even if they only care about the economy, as I'll explain in the next chapter.

FAT AND FOIE GRAS

Walking for half an hour a day, and reducing your carbohydrate load, is a very effective way to reduce blood pressure and cholesterol.[3,4] But why do that when the doctor can prescribe a pill? It's neither your fault, nor your doctor's. It's modern life and modern medicine, and it's not good. One 'statin' prescribed like jellybeans by doctors, and recommended by our governments for everyone, makes companies tens of billions in revenue every year. And doctors tell their patients to eat a miserable low-fat diet, when only 20 per cent of cholesterol comes from the diet, with 80 per cent produced by the liver. And why does the liver kick out bad cholesterol? Because it's sick from eating sugar, refined carbs and processed food! Putting any moral issues aside, when Gascon farmers want to induce huge fatty livers (for foie gras) in their big-bellied geese, they do not force-feed them fat; they force-feed them carbs, in the form of grains, to be precise. Think about that one! **Any Eurekas yet?!**

Would it not be sensible to stop the liver abuse caused by excess sugar, and eat plenty of healthy fats and fibre, rather than prescribe a pill that 50 per cent of people stop taking because of the side effects? And tell people honestly that the cholesterol story is far from sorted? That our brain is 60 per cent cholesterol, and that every cell in our body contains it, and that it is required for great health. I have rescued many friends in their eighth decade of life from the doctor-induced misery of a low-fat diet. Seen them miserable, eating salad, when they wanted a juicy big steak. This 'groupthink' is a toxic ideology and is both cruel and bonkers. Instead go for a walk and reduce the sugar, refined carbs and processed foods in your diet, and your cholesterol will do just fine. You can rate the harmfulness of carbs by this mantra: the higher the *refinement, the amount and the frequency*, the more they screw you over, damaging your liver and your metabolism and making you obese.

If you're still worried about cholesterol or not sure about statins, read Professor Malhotra's and Professor Lustig's brilliant overviews of statins and sugars respectively. You'll never look back. (You'll find the further reading at the end of the book). And then enjoy that steak fried in goose fat or lard and smothered in real butter, eaten with a pile of fibrous greens and a large glass of red. Delicious, bon appetit!

OUR JOURNEY TO THE PERFECT WEIGHT-LOSS SOLUTION

1. SOCIETAL CHANGE

We thought, if we looked at how society had changed over the last 50 years, would we find the correlation or causation there? And over time we certainly did. Changes in religious beliefs, smoking habits, divorce rates, single parenting and moving away from hometowns for work – these and many more environmental factors were all implicated. And what about the world's Blue Zones, where people not only enjoy a longer lifespan, but also a longer healthspan, free from illness, pills and doctors?

On this voyage of discovery, we learned that only a fool would think obesity had one cause and that the cure for it would be one single answer. Or that what works for one person would work equally well for another. We also learned there *is* most definitely an answer to both personal and societal obesity, which this book will teach you too. Individuals and society have changed and these changes are, in the main, likely irreversible. So, if we cannot un-change society, we need a solution that fits today's lifestyles, and preferably with some built-in future-proofing.

2. COMBINATION THERAPY

In our early years, Monique and I both worked in cancer therapy. So often, we waited with great expectancy for the next big breakthrough: the monoclonal antibody treatments and immunotherapy that have since revolutionised cancer care. But we remember those old cancer research units, where we spent our evenings mixing up the next day's chemo-therapy. And where almost none of the treatments were truly novel, but rather new combinations of old treatments. Much like the early days of HIV. Combination treatments that hit the sweet spot; combination treatments where the sum of the parts was greater than the whole. Monique and I began to realise that by combining traditional treatments with our modern understanding of hormones, we could provide a long-lasting solution to weight control. And most importantly, it wouldn't require fads, diet shakes and payments to diet companies. People would have the tools to put them back in charge of their own bodies. And you will discover too that combinations are the key to success.

3. FAT ADAPTING YOUR BODY

Latterly, we had been working on *fat adaptation* for endurance sports, like Ironman triathlon and ultra-running. Many athletes were, like the rest of society, and in a twentieth-century sort of way, completely attuned to pre-loading, fuelling and recovering on carbohydrates. Science said for many years that carbohydrate was the best fuel for endurance sport. Like everyone else, we had also been fuelling our endurance sports on carbohydrates.

But we had for many years been progressively, and somewhat intermittently, reducing refined carbohydrates in our own diet. And we knew the beneficial effects of omega-3 fats on life expectancy, and Monique had lectured on the gut microbiome. It seemed that if we brought all these things together, the sum of the parts may exceed the whole. But even applying these principles to ourselves, we had the same outcome: weight off for a while, then it all came back again, much to our frustration. We will cover why this happens in later chapters.

Like a hybrid car that runs on petrol or electricity, we too are a dual fuel system. Whereas our ancestors ran on dual fuels (fat and carbs), we run almost exclusively on carbs. Our modern bodies have been tuned to only burn carbs. Every meal, snack and drink has taught our bodies to be tuned to burning carbohydrates, and to lust after them: so called carb cravings. This happens not through the consumption of nutritious carbohydrate vegetables rich in fibre, but of flour- and sugar-based refined and super-refined carbohydrate food and drinks. Therefore, we need to *fat adapt* our body, to allow us to burn fat once again, and you'll soon know how to do this too.

You will also learn to control the hormones that *prevent* your body from burning fat to fuel your day-to-day activities. Just think about yesterday's meals. We often don't know what types of food were in the meal we ate. Imagine filling up a car and not caring or knowing what fuel you put in: petrol or diesel, who cares! That would hold up as reasonable evidence for insanity. Yet with food, not knowing what basic nutrients we're eating is normal. So, in the first part of the book we will empower you with the simple knowledge of basic foodstuffs – carbohydrates, fats and proteins. You will learn some shocking things along the way. Guaranteed!

The Diet Whisperer is about empowering you with knowledge to put you back in control.

4. THE CLOCK: FASTSPAN AND EATSPAN AND CIRCADIAN RHYTHM

Your body has a body clock, called the master clock, controlled by exposure to a good dollop of early morning light. This in turn controls the clocks in all your 30 trillion (or so) cells and organs. When you get your lifestyle and eating habits into a timely rhythm, you will have synchrony and this correlates with good health. And vice versa; bad irregular timings, poor morning light exposure, time zone changes, shift work and seasonal daylight-saving time changes play havoc with our clocks. This is of such importance we have included a chapter explaining it (see Chapter 13). I hope you love it as much as we do.

As we worked on the foods for fat adaptation, we also combined them with altered mealtimes. This stimulates new fat-burning pathways in the body. This is as old as the hills and can be traced back to Ancient Greek philosophers. The time between the last morsel to cross your lips at night and the first one in the morning gives us the name of the first meal of the day: breakfast, or break-the-fast! Timing is of fundamental importance to every aspect of a healthy life, as you will learn. We call this the *FastSpan®*. There are two other vitally important aspects to food and timing. Firstly, the time from the start of your first food of the day to the last morsel of the last meal, which we call the *EatSpan®*. And the second is the *number of meals* taken within the EatSpan.

5. WHY SNACK IS A VERY BAD NAME FOR A SMALL MEAL

At the Whisperer, there is no such thing as a snack; we call all snacks a meal, and from now on you should too. We call any drink other than water and black coffee/tea a meal too. The importance of this will become clear as your journey unwinds.

6. AUTOPHAGY IS A GREAT THING

It is extraordinary that most of the work on anti-ageing has a common theme: autophagy. Pronounced 'ort-off-a-gee'. It means the hoovering up of the ageing components within all our cells, by round fatty globules called lysosomes. To your cell it's like changing the old oil and replacing worn engine parts in the car. It's a process of renewal. Autophagy slows down with ageing and bits of large molecules and mitochondria (our cell's power stations) start to lie around in our cells, rather than getting vacuumed up. A bit like my study as I was writing this book, piles of paper building up around me; I will always reach a critical 'tipping point' where my efficiency slows down.

In ageing skin, the fibroblast cells that keep our skin smooth and elastic are getting stuffed up with their own products of intra-cellular life. In ageing, the renewal and repair processes that keep these cells fit and healthy are failing. The two most powerful tools to increase autophagy are fasting and exercise. We knew we needed to incorporate autophagy into any solution, and we'll show you how to too.

7. GUT BUGS

We now know that there is a wonderful battle that goes on in our gut every day, between bad bugs and good bugs. And we know that what we eat can empower the good guys or the bad guys. And that gut bugs change shifts at night, and they have a fantastic influence over our health, fitness and mood. Unsurprisingly, they have a big influence on our weight too, as you'll discover. They're important enough to get their own chapter (see Chapter 7).

THE SOLUTION

So, like in our old oncology jobs, we started to combine these factors into a twenty-first-century package that works. Flexible enough to respect the emotional, physiological and psychological differences between us. Flexible enough to allow us to err and regain control quickly. Like most men, I tend to go off-piste more than Monique, who is better-disciplined. Over the years as Monique and I worked on this nutrition plan, it became obvious there was always one common factor. One factor that controlled everything including us. *Our hormones; specifically, our nutritional and fat storage hormones.* That is how the Diet Whisperer was born. We will explain exactly the ways to bring all these factors together. By the end of the book, correcting your metabolism, cleansing your cells, getting to your target weight and improving your health will all be second nature.

You are joining thousands of people all around the world who have changed their lives through the Diet Whisperer Plans. But remember: do not change any aspect of your food until you have read Parts One and Two.

THE PHILOSOPHY OF THE DIET WHISPERER

This is quite simple. There is a mountain of information out there, but because of its medical tone, it doesn't pass easily to people without a scientific background. It's easy to lose the simple messages in medical jargon. This book, though, is here to help you to understand what you need to understand.

When you finish the book, you will have developed the skills needed to target your weight, get there, and stay there. We won't tell you what to eat at every hour of every day, or sell you ridiculous powdered drinks, or even make you eat horrid low-calorie foods. No, you will be able to go shopping, buy fresh food and know *what* you want to eat, and *when* it's best to eat it. You are the only person who knows which foods you like, and so as a principle it should be you who decides. You will learn to get back on track if you wander, and you will wander, if you're anything like me! You will be able to enjoy a drink and a meal with friends; you will value that time, and the joy of such occasions, without guilt. Your food plan must not be at the expense of a robust and healthy social life.

With our help, you will build a framework of nutrition, person-alised by you, specifically for you. You will then be able to furnish that framework and build your own healthy food plan. You may supplement parts of our plan with paleo, keto or vegan. Names don't matter. The principles of *'what food'*, and *'when food'* are the critical things to know. The most important thing is you understand what it is you're trying to achieve. Only then will you be on your new path for life; you will have joined the rest of us who can *whisper to our fat storage hormones.*

Welcome to the Diet Whisperer.

CHAPTER WHISPERINGS

- Before we learn to lose fat, we must learn what causes fat; only then will we succeed.
- Obesity leads to every department in the hospital.
- Science tells us that diets don't work; specifically, that they work for a while, then fail.
- Changes in lifestyle over the last 50 years have impacted on our weight.

- A combination of strategies is best for weight control.
- Fat adaptation is possible for both athletes and sedentary adults.
- EatSpan and FastSpan are critical to metabolic wellness and weight control.
- Increased autophagy slows ageing and ill-health; the whisperer plan increases autophagy.
- Our gut bugs, or gut microbiome, is a vital part of the overall solution.
- The common factor to metabolic wellness and weight loss is our nutritional hormones, and we teach you how to whisper them into your control.

Last reminder: please have some fun – and do the quiz on the website before you get into the book, so you can monitor how much you've learned by doing it again at the end; the results may surprise you!

Disclaimer

The Diet Whisperer represents our views and experiences and under no circumstance does it constitute medical advice. It was a movement born after leaving clinical medicine and has no connection whatsoever with the people or places we worked in. Although we are both medical doctors, we advise you to see your doctor before embarking on any advice in this book. And encourage your doctors to read it too! This plan is not suitable for children, but you will learn many principles that are. By working with your physician and the lessons in this book, there is a possibility you can reverse type 2 diabetes. If you have diabetes, take advice from your physician about hypoglycaemia and if you're on antihypertensive treatment about low blood pressure too. Your physician may have to supervise withdrawal of your medications to prevent excessive lowering of your blood pressure and/or blood glucose. If you have any medical condition, or psychological eating problems, you should not implement this, or any other nutrition plan, without discussing it with your doctor first. If your doctor refuses to help, no problem, you need a new doctor; move on. Assumptions are made in discussing hormones and physiology that changes and causes are not from underlying health conditions. We assume good health as the baseline for discussions.

PART ONE

THE ROAD TO OBESITY

PART ONE

THE ROAD TO OBESITY
The metabolic bus, en route to every hospital department

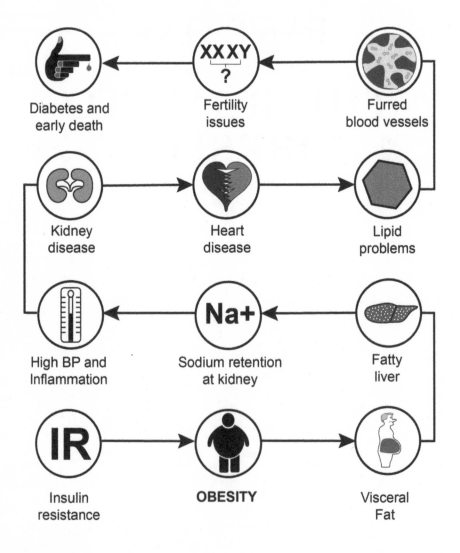

Figure. 1.1

1

THE OBESITY PANDEMIC

Thou seest I have more flesh than another man, and
therefore more frailty.

William Shakespeare, *Henry IV*

Obese people are not lazy people, and only lazy thinkers believe that.
Like most long-term conditions, obesity's origins lie in a complex
mixture of factors, a veritable minestrone soup. It is certainly a
mixture of nature and nurture. Nature is our genes, which are responsible for between 50 and 70 per cent of obesity. Nurture is responsible
for the rest.

In obesity, the influence of your genes increases as you get older. At
4 years old your genes have a smaller genetic influence on your actual
size (20 per cent) than they will at 35 years old (40 per cent) and by
the age of 80 (80 per cent).[1] You see, genetic influences change with
time, while environment influences change in both time and space. So
being born in Biafra in 1967 during the Nigerian civil war would be
very different from being born in the same place now. And, in turn, very
different from being born now in a small village in leafy Warwickshire.

While we cannot alter our genes, we have the power to influence
nurture. Nurture means environment, which means everything that
is not genetic. It means your place and date of birth, your school,
your job, where you live, pollution, pesticides, fertilisers, noise, stress,
wealth, education, your partner, your country, your habits, exercise
and fitness, what time you go to bed and rise, your food, how many
times a day you eat, snacking, alcohol, smoking, drugs, soft-drink
habits, the weather, the altitude of your home, the terrain you live
around, shift working, travel, methods of travel, occupation, your
hobbies, pets, neighbours, family, your social group or 'tribe', the

method of delivery when you were born, and the environmental factors your mother was exposed to while carrying you, including her diet. This is an important consideration if you are planning a family, and is called *epigenetics*. What you eat during pregnancy can and will affect what your child eats and what they weigh.

CHICKEN OR EGG

The temporal relationship between events means which comes first in time. The chicken or the egg, if you like. In the introduction I mentioned that we've all had this relationship wrong for 50 years. We thought that first came the fat, causing the imbalances in our body that then go on to make us ill with metabolic syndrome (see page 18 and Chapter 8), diabetes and all the consequences. Don't dwell too much on this for now; it will become clear as you progress through the book. We now know that the temporal relationship is opposite to what we thought for years, and that in fact metabolic changes come first, followed by obesity (Figure 1.1).

Critically, we now know what is *numero uno* in the chain of events leading to obesity! That is insulin resistance. And we use this as the main trigger to lose weight. Correct your metabolism, in particular insulin resistance, and the weight drops off, just as night follows day. And as over 88 per cent of Americans, obese or not, have at least one metabolic abnormality (as in any country where the Western Pattern Diet is predominant), trouble is down the road.

Here is where I introduce the concept of MONW, or metabolically obese normal weight, particularly prevalent in South Asians: often skinny with a tiny pot belly, and very prone to insulin resistance and other metabolic abnormalities and their serious consequences. At this point it is also worth mentioning another subgroup, which is a small number of people who are the opposite to MONW. This group, who are obese but metabolically normal, require periodic metabolic blood tests to know whether they remain metabolically normal or not. What we know is that these people will become ill and die prematurely from all causes.[2] But they are rare, so assuming you fall into this group, without appropriate tests, is unwise. And for simplicity, this book uses *obesity* to refer to people who are obese and metabolically abnormal, which is by far the biggest group; but it is equally applicable to our MONW friends.

GREAT NEWS

The really great news here is that there is some really great news. First, we can now diagnose dysfunctional metabolism early, and independent of your size. Second, when we do, we can turn it around, usually within one month of starting the *whisperer reset plan*. The longer-term and more severe your problems, the longer it takes. And third, when you turn around your metabolism, you get to feel a whole lot better straight away.

This whisperer plan is about putting you back in control. And not only that, but when your metabolism is healthy, your immunity is at its best, and boy do we know how important that is now. Bad metabolism equals poor immunity. During the peak of Covid-19, report after report showed that obese patients with metabolic diseases had a greater risk of severe disease or death. So, sorting your metabolism not only makes you feel better and lose weight, but gives a massive boost to your own immunity.

THE NOT-SO-FUN NUMBERS

Financially, we are drowning in obesity debt. In the USA, obesity alone is costing $150 billion a year. That money equates to the entire cost of the UK's National Health Service, which treats 70 million people free at the point of service, for one full year. Taking the last ten years' growth in health spend versus GDP and modelling it forwards, the US health budget will reach 50 per cent of GDP by 2035. Yes, I did say that: 50 per cent of GDP by 2035 (Figures 1.2 and 1.3).

Health spend as % of GDP

	50%	100%
AUSTRALIA	2052	2066
UK	2071	2087
USA	2035	2047

Figure 1.2. Graph of health spend when it reaches 50% of GDP and 100% of GDP for Australia, UK and US. All data extrapolated from each country's health spend growth versus GDP growth over the last 10 years and avoiding 2008.

	2021	2035	2045	2055	2065
AUS	11.59%	22.67%	36.62%	59.16%	95.56%
UK	5.39%	10.08%	15.08%	24.66%	38.58%
US	22.16%	50.36%	90.51%	162.7%	292.4%

Figure 1.3. Mathematical model based on the last 10 years' health spend and GDP growth. Health spend as a proportion of GDP up to 2065.

The US health budget will surpass its GDP in 2047. In very simple terms, unchecked healthcare costs will cause severe financial stress to the economies of countries where obesity follows the Western Pattern Diet. We need to find a fix. And we need it to start right now. Prevention through diet has never been more important.

We measure obesity in individuals by body mass index (BMI) (see Chapter 8). It is a calculation based on height and weight. It allows us to compare country to country quite well. It is less good for individuals because of differences in build types. You can calculate your own BMI on our website. Underweight is below 18.5, normal is 18.5 to 24.9, overweight is 25.0 to 29.9 and obese is over 30.0. So, in comparing countries we look at two figures. The first is the percentage of the population with a BMI >30, and the second is the average BMI for that country among all its people.

In 2021 more than 2.1 billion of our fellow humans are obese globally; 30 per cent of the world's population. Even booze-free countries in the Middle East (which do though, significantly, have a penchant for extra-sweet fizzy drinks) are piling on the pounds.

World Health Organization (WHO) reports show that globally 3 million deaths each year can be attributed to obesity and over 41 million preschool children are obese and will die prematurely. In American Samoa, a fantastical 74.6 per cent of the population are obese, and the population has an average BMI of 34.9. As comparators, the USA has a 36.2 per cent obesity rate, with the population average BMI 28.8; that is a staggering 119 million obese people. In the UK, the figures are 27.8 per cent obese, with an average Brit's BMI being 27.3. That equates to 19 million people with a BMI over 30.

The obesity epidemic is the cause of 'Peak Age', a term I have borrowed from the oil exploration and production industry; 'peak oil' represents that time when a tipping point in a well's production is reached and oil output starts to decrease. Some of the world's biggest life assurance companies (or rather their very smart actuaries) seem to agree with me that Peak Age is upon us. In other words, for the first time in 100 years, the rise in life expectancy is slowing, and I'm willing to bet will continue to fall. Life assurance companies are reducing their 'death contingencies', the financial provisions for coping with the pension demands of increasing life expectancy.

WHAT'S CHANGED IN THE WORLD?

As part of your journey and our journey, we have considered how our eating and other habits had changed over the last 50 years. We found many environmental changes. Church congregations are now smaller, and fasting rituals lost. The numbers smoking are fewer, and smoking is a powerful appetite suppressant. As a society, we spend more time in front of the television and value the dining table less. We work longer hours and divorce rates are up. We cook less than previous generations; much food is purchased pre-prepared, ready for nuking in the microwave. Markets struggle as supermarkets flourish. There are new aisles of food wrapped in cardboard and plastic, perfect for dumping in the ocean. Cereal-makers bring us a plethora of boxed breakfasts and the cooked full English is on the wane. Lard and butter have been replaced by pro-inflammatory seed cooking oils and margarine. And, as you will learn, by the advent of hideous foods like low-fat yoghurts.

We have cola and other similar fizzy drinks in ever larger bottles, for ever larger kids. And the sugars in fruit juices are just as lethal, as you'll discover.

Cars are used more and bicycles less; but how much influence does exercise have on our weight anyway, particularly weight loss? We know that in the world's Blue Zones, where people are healthy and live longest, their exercise is incidental to life, and they do not use gyms. We also know that there is a U-shaped curve with an optimum amount of exercise per day – the amount that people in Blue Zones exercise. And being fitter does not necessarily mean healthier, particularly if you're doing long and hard stuff.

Our societies have embraced multiculturalism, and the choice of foods available has changed, for the better. Forget the spice routes: East and South Asian food is now available on every high street. Capitalism has made us materially richer but has also befuddled our minds, giving us too much choice of things like shoes as well as food.[3] Modern life makes us travel more and sleep less. Time zones are regularly crossed. Morning larks are in the majority, and can therefore bully the night owls into waking, arising and working at a time that is neither natural nor healthy for them. We have the nonsense of daylight saving time, associated with a surge each year in heart attack numbers.[4] Fast food outlets have sprung up in every city in the world. And these outlets are commoner in poorer areas, supermarkets scarcer.

Since 1961, we have seen the industrialisation of bread production, with additional preservatives, modern wheats, and homogenous gluten. (The French baguette is a notable exception that not only tastes good, but is reassuringly stale by lunchtime. And the French are an exception too, with high-fat diets and the second lowest deaths from heart disease worldwide: this is known as the French paradox.)

We have seen individual behaviour change too. During my English upbringing, no snacks between meals or fizzy drinks were ever allowed. We ate wholesome home-cooked food, usually meat and two vegetables. We all had great appetites, caused by ghrelin, our hunger hormone. Our evening meal was taken early. We were taught to eat slowly and chew our food well. It contained all the macro-nutrients – never any fear of fat – and much fibrous greens. Later we would eat toast spread with cold beef dripping for supper. And we were all fit and thin.

OBESITY, VISCERAL FAT AND METABOLIC SYNDROME

Metabolic syndrome is a condition that occurs silently without symptoms and in those who are slim as well as overweight people. If you have it, you must find out, as it can be reversed by changing your environment, most importantly your diet. And the sooner you discover it, the quicker you'll recover. It is a cluster of conditions: visceral fat (the fat unseen inside your abdomen), high blood pressure (hypertension), high blood sugar (glucose), high triglycerides (TG) and high bad cholesterol (LDL-C). If you are obese, you have an 80 per cent chance of visceral fat and metabolic syndrome. Metabolic syndrome is associated with just about every non-infectious chronic condition, from arthritis and cancer to pregnancy problems, dementia and blindness. Its causes, diagnosis and consequences are discussed in detail in Chapter 8.

THE TWO CARBOHYDRATE REVOLUTIONS

Our diets changed 12,000 years ago, with the onset of agriculture and the *first carbohydrate revolution*. We learned how to cultivate wheat and from the flour (starch) made delicious foods such as bread and pasta. Over the last 100 years, our diets have transformed even more radically, as the carbohydrates flour, starch and sugar were combined to make cakes, pastries and doughnuts: the *second carbohydrate revolution*. The introduction of refined carbohydrates followed by super-refined carbohydrates has adversely impacted our health (more in Chapter 4). Remember, these carbs' negative impact on you increases with *refinement, amount and frequency*.

We have gone from being creatures whose lives depended on food availability to being creatures who are being killed by excess food. The changes have happened too quickly to allow us to evolve and adapt. Some argue that we may have seen some adaptation to the first carbohydrate revolution, but it would be impossible for our bodies to have adapted of the 50-times carb loading of the last 100 years. We did not evolve to eat super-refined carbohydrates. We evolved over thousands of years to conserve energy; we had to, as food was scarce. In these modern times of plenty, we store too much energy as fat, making us ill and obese.

EAT MORE, TAKE PILLS

We are at the mercy and whim of large corporate companies, or Big Food, who fill our lives with adverts for foods we ill need. We are awash with messages to eat more, eat three meals a day and then snack in between. Most people now believe that missing a meal is bad or, even worse, dangerous. Overeating and eating junk food is the new normal. We are rewarded with sugar highs, a compulsive feeling that needs to be repeated again and again. Our food environment has departed hugely from our ancestors' and our hormones, while perfectly designed to keep us healthy in the past, are now in a maelstrom of chaos (see Chapter 10).

We move less than we did. Many are socially isolated and lonely. Antidepressants are rife, but we show scant regard to tryptophan in our diet, the precursor of serotonin, our happy hormone. We overlook our microbiome's influence over serotonin production. We treat our microbiome like a weed patch rather than a beautiful cottage garden (see Chapter 7 for more on the microbiome).

In the recent past we have lost 20 per cent of our sleep time.[5] We show indifference to it and to the sleep hygiene needed to ensure a good sleep cycle, even though sleep is essential for our bodily repair, restoration and health (see Chapter 13).

Our environmental, lifestyle and dietary changes have resulted in a pandemic of non-communicable (infectious) diseases: metabolic syndrome, cancer, diabetes and cardiovascular disease and all their consequences. Rates of obesity are soaring and obesity is associated with poor metabolic health and a plethora of non-communicable diseases. And worryingly, even non-obese people are suffering poor metabolic health, followed by disease (see Chapter 8).

HOSPITAL STAFF

Hospital staff, too, simply cannot cope with the increase in workload. Doctors and nurses are retiring earlier.[6] Burnout is extremely common, and as more medical professionals retire early, the remaining pool becomes depleted of knowledge and experience, and standards fall, with more complaints and with more burnout; and so the cycle repeats. Our hospitals will be short of staff and skills and stuffed full of people with obesity-related diseases and people with metabolic abnormalities. The rest of us will have nowhere to go. Unchecked, this rather dystopian picture will be upon us in the next decade. Frightening!

CORPORATE FOOD SCIENCE

Big Food multinationals quest only for profit. They work to find the 'bliss point' for our taste buds; the perfect mix of salt, sugar and fat. Your fast food tasting great is not a coincidence; it's made to be like that. For the record, I'm pro-business, pro-profit and for people's freedom to choose. But when any business supplies a product that is addictive and is killing millions of people, we have a serious problem. When we had a similar problem with cigarettes, our governments did something about it.

Our hormones have been turned into a confused soup by the rubbish that passes our lips. We can no longer taste sweet, because we have 50 times as much sugar in our diet than is safe, and our hormones can't tell us when we are full.[7,8] Twelve bags of sugar (24 pounds) is the recommended annual *maximum* sugar consumption in the US; but annual average sugar consumption is 150 pounds, or 1.5 bags per week. That's the equivalent of a wheelbarrow-load each year, or in honey terms, one year's work for 6 hives and 300,000 busy bees.

OBESITY IS CONTAGIOUS

We know this in our house and see it everywhere we travel. On asking a friend overseas how he was doing, he replied that he and his wife were happily getting fatter together. Office colleagues also tend to get fat together. We know that couples share common good gut bugs, which are associated with leaner bodies (see Chapter 7). We also know that people who are obese have a lower diversity of gut bugs (again, see Chapter 7) and more of the bad guys. And we don't just share our skin microbiota with our pets; they also lower our stress hormones, reducing our obesity factors; so don't shoot the cat.

It is a great idea to whisper to your hormones in a group, or as a couple, because you can learn and build together. There are many lessons in this book that will make your whole family much, much healthier, mentally as well as physically. That's why we recommend setting up Diet Whisperer groups locally, where you can all help each other. And keeping a food diary or journal can be a great motivator too.

WHAT IS DIET WHISPERING?

Diet whispering is learning to whisper to your hormones. Not only will you feel so much better straight away, but you'll be back in charge. You will have total control of your weight, as well as seeing instant improvements in your physical and mental wellness.

You will learn which hormones cause obesity and why (see Chapters 8 and 10). And that they are canny, and hard to fool. If you fight them, they will fight back and win, easily and convincingly. And if you fail to look after them, they will kill you slowly and mercilessly.

In Aesop's fable, 'The North Wind and the Sun', the sun challenges the wind to a competition to remove a man's coat. The wind uses force and the sun persuasion. And the sun wins, of course. So, just like the fable, to beat our hormones we use whispering, nudging and the art of persuasion. In doing so, we can recreate our senses of hunger and satiety, and feel better and better as our metabolism improves and the pounds fall away.

CHAPTER WHISPERINGS

- Obesity is not overeating and laziness; believing this is lazy thinking.
- Obesity and long-term medical conditions are a mixture of nature and nurture.
- The obesity pandemic is a truly global phenomenon.
- We measure total body fat by BMI.
- BMI has limitations in individuals due to racial differences and build types.
- Metabolic syndrome leads to long-term diseases and premature death.
- Obesity affects 40 million preschool children globally.
- Calorie restriction and exercise do not cause a sustained reduction in obesity.
- Corporate food scientists, know how to create the 'bliss point' for taste.
- Genetic factors play a part, and one that increases throughout life, but we can still win the battle.
- Obesity is contagious and people do better when they form diet whisperer groups.
- Most 'fad' diets cause a clash between the dieter and their hormones; and the hormones always win. Every single time.

2

WHAT IS FOOD?

Der Meunsch ist was er isst. (A man is what he eats).
Ludwig Feuerbach, 1862

This chapter and the next three are the foundations of the whisperer plan. If 'man is what he eats', he can only know what he is if he knows what he eats. And therein lies one of our fundamentals. A fundamental part of metabolic illness and obesity is not knowing exactly what our food is made from. One of the things this book will do is to make it possible for you to not only know this, but also teach these essential skills to your family, children, or grandchildren. Or – dare I suggest – your parents; science informs us that there is no age in life where exercise and nutrition cannot make a positive difference to health and wellbeing.

Let's dive head-first into what food is. We know that we have foods that we like and foods we find boring. What we have to do in any food or nutrition plan is to ensure that what we eat is enjoyable. This is one of the myriad reasons why all diets have a quick win and then long-term failure. We're human and we love the ritual of eating and what is put before us. So, might I offer this as a guiding principle: I'm not going to suggest you eat things you don't like. But I am going to suggest that to lose weight, and maintain that loss, we do need to invest a small amount of time in the food chapters here. Unless we know what it is that we're buying, preparing and eating, we cannot win this battle, let alone the war.

WHAT IS A MEAL?

For the purposes of this book, and hopefully your future thinking, it is important to know what *does not* constitute a meal: unsweetened black coffee, black tea, green tea, unsweetened herbal tea and water, still or sparkling. It will become clear why, from your fat storage hormones' perspective, everything else is food. So, tea or coffee with milk is food.

In this book, when any food, and I do mean *any* food, passes your lips it constitutes a meal. So, one digestive biscuit with your elevenses, or at bedtime with your cocoa, is a meal. Even on its own, the cocoa is a meal.

We do not use the term snack. Snack implies a tiny little something that is not really important in the larger scheme of things. Your fat storage hormones don't see it that way. And as you learn to control these hormones, you will come to see it that way too. For the sake of clarity, we use the terms breakfast, lunch and supper.

MACRONUTRIENTS AND MICRONUTRIENTS

We know that our foods are a mixture of all sorts of things. It is vital to understand the differences. Simply, macronutrients are big nutrients that we need a lot of, compared to micro, or small, nutrients that we need in small amounts. Water is also a vital macronutrient but, accepting we need 4–6 pints (2–3 litres) per day, we'll put that to one side for now.

Macronutrients is the medical name for the three groups of food you already know: carbohydrates, fats and proteins. I'm going to expand on these in the next three chapters, as they are key to your success, but briefly:

1. **Carbohydrates** are also known as carbs or CHO. You will come across all these terms and they mean the same thing. When carbohydrates travel around the body in the blood, it is in the form of blood sugar, more formally referred to as blood glucose. I shall use the term blood glucose.

2. **Fats** we all have a feel for, if we've seen meat with fat on it. There are also many other sources of fats, including vegetables, as we'll see below. It is a terrible mistake to think fat = bad; from

the mainstream media to politicians and your own family doctor, we have all been indoctrinated with this, but you will soon learn why it is not true.

3. **Proteins** are sourced from both animals, in the form of lean meat or fish and dairy products, and vegetables like chickpeas, lentils, nuts and seeds.

And let me say this once only: the human body powers itself by electron transfer, and is not a school bomb calorimeter. There is no fire! It is therefore not about the calories you eat, but the *type* of food (which macronutrient) and the *timing* of the food. In turn these two very important factors will decide, via your fat storage hormones, what effect the food has, that is, whether it will be used for energy or stored as (mainly) fat. Never trust anyone who says a calorie is a calorie, or calories in = calories out, and that that will cause long-term weight loss. If you take the exact same daily food and eat it as one meal or ten meals, the effects on fat storage will be profoundly different. And if you eat a certain number of calories in fat and the same in carbs, the fat storage will be radically different too.

Micronutrients are the smaller things necessary in our diet in lesser amounts. We split micronutrients into two groups.

1. Minerals, for example, calcium, magnesium, selenium, zinc, iron and iodine, which help maintain healthy bones, teeth, immune system, nerves, blood cells and hormones.
2. Vitamins. The first four are stored in fats and the body can go for periods without them. They are known as the fat-soluble vitamins: A, D, E and K. The water-soluble vitamins, which are easily washed from the body in urine, need frequent top-ups as we cannot store them. These are B1, B2, B3, B6, B7, B12 and folate. And last but not least, vitamin C.

NUTRIENT PROFILING: CALORIE DENSITY AND NUTRIENT DENSITY

These are ways of describing the density of calories (energy), or the density of nutrients, in a standard amount of food. In other words, how much energy we get per portion or how many nutrients we get per portion. Macronutrients provide us with our energy measured in calories. You can think of macronutrients as having a 'calorie density': a certain number of calories per gram of food. Carbohydrates' calorie density is 4 calories per gram, fats' is 9 calories per gram and protein's 4 calories per gram. (But we mustn't let this put you off dietary fats, as you will discover.)

Micronutrients provide us with all the things we need to stay alive. The things that allow other foods to be digested, cells walls to remain healthy, vitamins and enzymes to be created or repaired, our bones to grow, or allow us to maintain good eyesight and healthy eyes. Quite simply, without them we become ill and die prematurely so they are vitally important. They can be measured by comparing the number of nutrients with the calorific value or the weight of the foodstuff, for example, calories per 100 grams.

We need to eat less food, but make sure we get all the right micro-nutrients for development, health and life. This comes from eating nutritionally dense foods. We also need to consume less food that is packed with calories but of little or no nutrient benefit: low-nutrient-density foods. These are also known as 'empty calories', or called 'calorie-dense, nutrient-poor'. A sugar cube is the ultimate empty calorie; it has lots of calories, but not one essential nutrient for the body. And we're all sensible enough not to go munching sugar cubes. Another example is carbonated soft drinks (CSDs), or fizzy drinks. Alas, we have much learning ahead about these time-bombs. Nutritionally dense foods are foods that give you all your good nutrients in fewer calories. Examples are:

- Ocean: Salmon, shellfish, sardines, mackerel, tuna and seaweed.
- Land: Beef, lamb, venison that are grass-fed and grass-finished. 'Lesser' cuts like brisket and oxtail are even more nutritionally dense than leaner cuts, the most dense being liver. Eggs are great too.
- Plants, fruits and berries: whole fruits and superfoods like kale, cooked spinach and marsh samphire. Potato skins are also rich in cellulose fibre.
- Herbs and spices, including garlic.

Calorie-dense, nutrient-poor foods are for treats when weight is in the stable phase, but should be avoided altogether for maximum weight reduction in the reducing phase. Examples of these are:

- Refined carbohydrates: pastries, pizza, pasta, rice, bread and potato. Potato is a bit of a mixed bag; the skin is highly nutritious because of its fibre. The white pulp falls into the refined category, as it is starch.
- Super-refined carbohydrates: fizzy drinks, biscuits, muffins.
- Alcohol: especially sweet wines, but also beers, other wines – and watch those sugary mixers!

Now, I'm the last one to spoil the fun. Socialising is important for health, and I'm not judgemental on such matters. But you need the facts! If you want to cook breads, chapatis or pizza bases, look at ancient flour like emmer or einkorn. Modern flour's homogeneity is part of its problem. When you are in your stable phase, make these a treat and when you do, eat them with great joy.

ALCOHOL

Alcohol is not a macronutrient but it gets a special mention here. For many people drinking is a big part of life, and we all know that it is associated with a number of health problems – and a few health benefits.

So, what is alcohol? Essentially it is a toxin, one which our liver kindly sorts out for us. The problem is that while the liver is sorting out the booze it is preoccupied. It is possible to drink and diet, but the best thing is to cut out the drink until you reach your target weight. If that won't work for you, then look at what you drink and find out the carb content of your favourite tipple. Mine is a long vodka with zero carbs. I add sparkling water to the vodka with ice, a slice of cucumber and five drops of Angostura bitters. Delicious. Other drinks that you can have are red wine, dry white wine and shorts. Mixers can be 'diet' mixers that have zero carbs. The real problems with alcohol and losing weight are that it turns off your fat burn, and any carb content will make your daily carb count climb. It also turns off the sensible part of your brain and you might find yourself heading for the pizza house! My general advice is to stop until you achieve your target weight. Habits take about six weeks to break, so it might be your opportunity to change your lifestyle while also shifting the pounds.

CHAPTER WHISPERINGS

- Understanding food is the foundation to building your diet whisperer house.
- Diet whisperers do not use the word snack; it's a meal.
- Water, black coffee and tea are the only non-meals.
- Food consists of macronutrients or micronutrients.
- Macronutrients are carbohydrates, fats and proteins.
- Micronutrients are our minerals and vitamins.
- Nutrient profiling gives us the density of food calories or food nutrients.
- In human nutrition a calorie is not a calorie
- High nutritional density is great.
- Low-nutrient-density foods are to be avoided during weight loss.
- Low-nutrient-density foods can be intermittent treats after weight loss.
- Alcohol is best avoided during the loss stage, as it slows fat loss.

3

YOUR GUT MADE SIMPLE

Things sweet to taste, prove in digestion sour.
William Shakespeare, *Richard II*

Of course, we all benefit from knowing how our body works, but rather than try to make you the next Christiaan Barnard, I'll stick to the relevant bits that you *need* to know; the where and how of food absorption.

FOOD AND THE ALIMENTARY CANAL

That's the medical name for the sewage pipe that goes through you and connects your mouth to your anus. At the bottom end is a ring of muscle called the anal sphincter; and a very clever fellow it is too. Thankfully, it retains its muscle tone while we sleep. Mercifully, it can differentiate between a fart and solids. (Farting, while socially unacceptable, is a sign of a healthy diet and fermenting microbiome.) So, there we have it. There is a sphincter at the top that allows you to pout your lips for a selfie, and one at the bottom that keeps your trousers clean.

CLEAN AND DIRTY

Get poop in your bloodstream and you're dead. And you don't need a doctor to tell you that. And this is an important concept. Food turns into poop as it travels down your gut. The *inside* of your gut is classed as *outside* of the body. Imagine holding a hosepipe as water passes through it – your hand stays dry. That's the same with the bowel (also called the gut, intestine or alimentary canal). Food goes in at the top, some clever stuff happens, and poop emerges at the bottom.

LEAKY GUT

Between each cell in our bowel are special seals, called 'tight-junctions'. These prevent communication between the content of the bowel and our body or blood. When they fail, tiny amounts of proteins from the gut can enter the bloodstream. This drives our immune system crazy, and it charges around in a high state of alert, all day every day. This is the basis of many autoimmune diseases. Sort out your 'leaky gut', through the right foods and fibre, and the problem either doesn't occur, or goes away! Leaky gut is also associated with other physical and mental conditions.

SMALL INTESTINE

At the top you have a straight tube that goes to your stomach, called the oesophagus. Your stomach is a muscular bag that mixes chewed food with stomach acid and then squeezes it out into the next pipe, your small intestine. This is made up of three parts, the duodenum, the jejunum and the ileum (Figure 3.1). It is here that the food is broken down further by digestive enzymes and *absorbed* into your blood (see below). The small bowel is 1 inch (2.5 cm) in diameter and 10 feet (3 metres) long. It ends where it joins the large intestine. Diseases of the small intestine include Crohn's disease, ulcers, coeliac disease and small intestine bacterial overgrowth (SIBO). The gut wall has muscle fibres that gently squeeze the food along, a propelling process known as peristalsis. At the top of the small gut, digestive juices enter from the gall bladder and the pancreas. As your food passes though it emerges into the next pipe, the large intestine.

LARGE INTESTINE

After your food is digested, and some nutrients have been absorbed from the small bowel into your blood, the remnants emerge into the large bowel, just above the right groin. At this junction of small and large gut lies your appendix (or your appendectomy scar!). Diseases of the large intestine (or large bowel) include constipation, irritable bowel syndrome (IBS), diarrhoea and ulcerative colitis. The large bowel is 3 inches (7.5 cm) in diameter and 5 feet (1.5 metres) long. It passes up your right flank, then horizontally over to your left just under your ribs, down the left flank into your rectum, where the poop is in a holding pattern until air traffic control allows it to touch down in

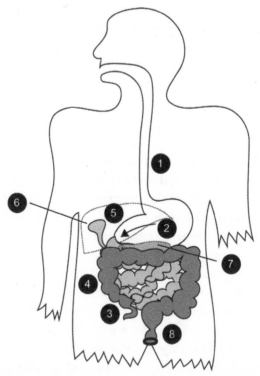

Figure 3.1. 1: Food pipe or oesophagus. 2: Stomach emptying into light grey small intestine (arrow). 3: Caecum and appendix where small intestine empties into large bowel. 4: Colon or large gut. 5: Liver. 6: Gall bladder opening into smalll intestine. 7: Pancreas opening into small intestine. 8: Rectum and anus. Gut bugs are found from the mouth to the anus, but mainly in the colon.

the pan. In Germany, their bogs have an inspection shelf, disconcerting to any English speaker. In France until just a few years ago it was two footplates with a hole in the middle of the ground: difficult enough when sober. In the Middle East some sort of jet spray is preferred to paper and in Greece, the birthplace of democracy, the outlet pipe capacity allows for liquids and solids but not paper, which must be deposited in a bag. In Japan, they now have computerised versions that flash lights, warm the seat and play music while your under-carriage gets a jet wash, then a blow-dry. Make up your own mind.

The main 'physical' function of the large bowel is manufacturing poop from the remnants of digestion. It does so by absorbing much of the water out of it. But our bowels also contain 38 trillion bugs, collectively called the microbiome. Such is the importance of the microbiome to every aspect of human life, including metabolism, obesity and mood, that we have dedicated a whole chapter (see

Chapter 7) to it. If you learn one thing from this book, let it be to look after your microbiome. Treat it like your most beloved cottage garden; toil for it, fight for it, and treat it with tender loving care. As the book progresses you will realise how to achieve this, with *what* food and *when* food.

DIGESTION

Macronutrients as eaten cannot be absorbed. They would just pass through us. We chew our food as the first process of breaking it down. It then gets an acid wash in the stomach and is churned around into a nutrient-rich mixture of the macronutrients, carbs, proteins and fats. The stomach then churns it again and mulches it, mixes it with enzyme-rich juices from your stomach and pancreas and like a sausage machine squeezes the mush into the small intestine, where *absorption* of nutrients occurs. Before absorption can occur, the enzymes break those strings of nutritional pearls into their constituent parts (Figure 4.2, Figure 5.1, Figure 6.1). So, carbs are broken down into mono and disaccharides; one or two sugar units (more in Chapter 4). Fats and proteins are similarly broken down into their constituent units, fatty acids and amino acids respectively (see Chapters 5 and 6).

Their next obstacle to reaching our bloodstream is the bowel wall. If we simply had holes though our bowel wall into our blood, or vice versa, infection would pass from one to the other.

This mashing up and breaking down of food into constituent parts, or macronutrient units, is to allow absorption.

ABSORPTION

The small bowel is surrounded by a plethora of blood vessels waiting to transport our digested food away to the liver, our food processing plant. When Harry Potter[1] was waiting for the *Hogwarts Express*, he had to get to platform 9¾, which lay between platforms 9 and 10 at London's King's Cross railway station. He did so by walking through the brick wall. And the secret here is that as he passed through, the wall stayed intact. While many readers thought this magical, most doctors would have recognised it as the normal, yet miraculous way macronutrients move from the bowel, through the bowel wall and into the blood. The bowel is our platform 9¾, the wall of which our macronutrients must cross, to catch the blood express, which will take them not to Hogwarts but to the liver for processing. If you perforate your bowel and its contents enter the surrounding sterile peritoneum, resulting in peritonitis, there is a 30 per cent risk of death. And that's in the very best hospitals in the world. So, absorption must occur in the presence of an intact, bacteria-proofed, bowel wall.

The rules for how much *absorption* takes place are very simple:

1. The longer your small intestine, the more absorption of macro-nutrients takes place.
2. Surface area is a factor; the greater the contact with the gut wall, the more absorption of macronutrients takes place, which is why we have ridges and villi (finger-like projections) that make the gut wall's surface area some 600 times that of a tennis court.
3. The speed at which food passes through is also a factor; the more slowly it passes, the more absorption of macronutrients take place.
4. The presence of fibre (solid and liquid types; see Chapter 4) surrounds food, and liquid types line the gut wall and speed up transit, thereby reducing absorption of macronutrients. So orange juice causes a sugar rush, which is reduced massively by the fibre when the whole fruit is eaten instead.

SYNERGISTIC FOODS

This is where one or more foods work to aid the absorption or effects of another. These foods combined get a greater nutrient absorption or effect than they would alone. Examples are tomatoes and broccoli; tomatoes peel-on and olive oil; turmeric and black pepper; apples and their peel; fruits combined like a fruit salad; and garlic and fish.

Also, remember when you look at a food label, with the information of 'x' grams per 100 grams, although that is the amount you will eat and digest it may be very different from the amount you *absorb* into your blood, the amount that is nutritionally available.

ANTAGONISTIC FOODS

This is where one or more foods work against the absorption or effects of another, like vitamin A and vitamin D, and vitamin D and certain anticoagulants.

CHAPTER WHISPERINGS

- From mouth to anus is our alimentary canal or gut.
- The gut has friendly bugs called our microbiome.
- Digestion breaks down our food into its constituent 'pearls' or 'units'.
- Only when a food is absorbed will it be available for nutrition.
- The tiny macronutrients are absorbed across the gut wall into our blood.
- Nutrients may be synergistic or antagonistic to each other.

4

CARBOHYDRATES

La plus belle des ruses du diable est de vous persuader qu'il n'existe pas. (The devil's finest trick is to persuade you that he does not exist.)

Charles Baudelaire, *Paris Spleen*

Many good nutrition books state that carbohydrates are the only *non-essential* macronutrient for human nutrition, albeit the one we eat the most of. And I understand that, because in an old-fashioned sense our body's macronutrient metabolism can make everything we need to survive from fats and proteins. In my medical school days, biochemistry taught us that we can live on meat or fish alone; both contain fats as well as lean protein and water. But you must eat much of it raw, and eat the whole animal – and, as was tradition among groups including Inuits and indigenous Australians, the stomach's contents! Any glucose the body requires can be manufactured from those fats and proteins by the liver (see Chapter 12).

But there is one missing factor. We need our gut bugs to be healthy for us to be healthy. And these healthy gut bugs feed largely on fibre from indigestible carbohydrates. So, as we are unlikely to find feet, hooves and stomach contents to our liking, we definitely do need *unrefined* carbohydrate fibre in our diet, as I shall explain below and in Chapter 7.

However, to clarify, *refined* and *super-refined* carbohydrates are definitely not required for human health. And super-refined carbs are simply harmful. They give our bodies a shapeless form; they round the edges in a way you'll learn to notice if you observe others on refined and super-refined carbohydrate diets. Arms lose their shape and become featureless; lovely arms are not built on carbs! The carbohydrate arms, legs, neck, belly, face and bum; I can recognise carbohydrate overload at 100 paces. And soon you will too.

Refined and super-refined carbohydrates are directly or indirectly associated with obesity, cancer, metabolic syndrome, central nervous system diseases, heart disease, dementia, chronic inflammatory conditions, childhood obesity and childhood allergies. In fact, they are linked to just about every non-communicable disease of our modern era. Refined and super-refined carbohydrates change our gut bugs, feeding the bad bugs and poisoning the good ones. Some carbohydrates are our most dangerous macronutrient; accordingly, we will spend a few pages covering their most important and deadly aspects.

Over the years, terminology has muddied the waters; but as we shall see, carbohydrates are in fact extremely easy to understand. Carbohydrate means 'carbon and water', and that is what they are made of (in chemical terms C, H and O). The first concept about carbs is to look around you. Trees, plants, bushes, flowers, all those things in the vegetable patch, and your back lawn are all carbohydrates. While a lawnmower is more efficient than your teeth at trimming the back lawn, and a giraffe better at chewing through the thorns, twigs and leaves of the mimosa tree, these are nevertheless carbs. They're all around us; in our beautiful world they are truly ubiquitous.

Our early human ancestors foraged for carbs. Imagine having to find all your vegetables in the wild. To complement your meat or fish, you would pick fruits, seeds or tree nuts, rather than simply opening a packet from the supermarket and devouring the lot. After 190,000 years of doing this very successfully, human eating habits went through the two carbohydrate revolutions outlined in Chapter 1.

The First Carbohydrate Revolution: 12,000 Years Ago

The Fertile Crescent of the Levant lies between the Persian Gulf and the Eastern Mediterranean, curling around Northern Syria (Figure 4.1). Here the Neolithic or agricultural revolution took place, with domestication of animals, planting of large-scale crops and even granary stores and flour. This was when the first big increase in human carbohydrate consumption occurred. It was the first appearance of refined carbohydrates from flour (starch) in the human diet. Traditional bread (without added sugar) and pasta came from flour (starch), while rice and potatoes grow as starches.

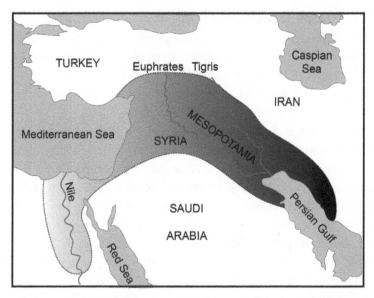

Figure 4.1. The Fertile Crescent in the eastern Mediterranean was the birthplace of agriculture. From there, cultivation techniques spread across the entire world.

The Second Carbohydrate Revolution: 100 Years Ago

This is the one that we're in the midst of now. In the last 100 years, we have increased one type of carbohydrate in our diet over 50-fold: the super-refined carbohydrate. Again, another first for the human body was the addition of sugar to flour to make food. Think cakes, biscuits, energy bars, fizzy drinks and modern bread.

Timescale of the carb problem

Think of it this way; if we plot man's existence of 190,000 years on a scale of 100 years, we would have seen the *first carbohydrate revolution* 5 years ago. The *second carbohydrate revolution*, our current super-refined carb rush, would have begun just 18 days ago! Houston, we have a problem; and it doesn't take Cape Canaveral's boffins to work out that the problem is our consumption of refined and super-refined carbs in particular. Carbohydrates are our commonest food, known as our staples. They are energy-dense, nutrient-poor foods and were useful in times gone by to replenish the energy lost from manually tilling the fields.

WHAT IS A CARBOHYDRATE?

Think of a string of pearls. The pearls are units of sugar, the commonest of which we encounter being glucose, fructose and galactose (Figure 4.2). When we string them together, the 'string' connecting each sugar unit is called a 'bond'. And bonds can be cut by 'tiny scissors' called enzymes present in our gut.

Glucose 'strings' found in plants are called starch or cellulose. We can digest starch as our gut has the necessary enzymes (essentially scissors) to cut the starch into tiny sugar units that can be absorbed. Once absorbed, the sugars are re-strung in the liver as human starch, called glycogen.

Starch and cellulose have one important difference: the bonds between the glucose units are different. In starch there is an *alpha bond*, but in cellulose there is a *beta bond*. Humans have no gut enzyme for the beta bond, which *is* found in the guts of rabbits, locusts, deer and other ruminants including giraffes.

When glucose chains in cellulose link up with other chains, they eventually make structures like a cellulose leaf, like lettuce, grass, or eventually a tree. Cellulose is broken down to glucose when eaten by animals, but not by humans. Interestingly, some of our gut bugs (see Chapter 7) *do have* the cellulase enzyme necessary to break down cellulose, for personal use!

Starch and cellulose

So, starches are the digestible part of fruit and vegetables, and cellulose the indigestible part. And all foods can be put on a scale. A sugar cube, which needs no digestion and is rapidly absorbed, would be at one end. Further along you'll find a potato, which has a starch pulp but some cellulose in the skin. And so on. At the other end of the scale we have green vegetables, like runner beans and kale, which are mainly indigestible cellulose, also called fibre or roughage.

Best for health are vegetables high in cellulose, which pass undigested into the large gut as *fibre*. So, for any food, we need to know the starch content, the sugar content and the fibre content. *Net carbs* is a concept you will become familiar with – it is the part of the food that we can digest. *Net carbs* are calculated as total carbs, *minus* the fibre.

Carb bonds that break easily we call *quickly digesting* carbs. Any carbohydrate that breaks easily in our guts can then be absorbed rapidly into our bloodstream.

SINGLE SUGAR = MONOSACCHARIDE

GLUCOSE

FRUCTOSE

GALACTOSE

TWO SUGARS = DISACCHARIDE

TABLE SUGAR: SUCROSE

MILK: LACTOSE = 2—8% OF MILK

THOUSANDS OF SUGARS = POLYSACCHARIDE

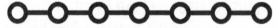

GLYCOGEN, STARCH AND CELLULOSE

Figure 4.2. Carbohydrates are made up from chains of sugar molecules, connected by special alpha bonds. In starch, these are enzymatically broken down during digestion, absorbed into the blood and remade for storage in the body in the form of branched glycogen. Glycogen is found in skeletal muscle (70%) and liver (30%). Cellulose is not digestable because of the beta bonds, the enzymes for which we do not have, but which is present in cows, sheep deer and others.

Refined carbs are those foods with naturally occurring starches (potatoes, rice), and those made from wheat grasses (flour, pasta, bread). These are long chains of glucose (only), that can be rapidly broken down into glucose and absorbed. Starch has three significant properties:

1. It is a chain of glucose-*only* 'pearls'.
2. These glucose pearls are joined by 'bonds' and we have enzymes that 'cut' them into single glucose units for absorption.
3. The branching of the chains makes them more bioavailable (see page 42).

Super-refined carbs are manufactured processed foods like sweets, fruit juices, fizzy drinks, muffins, shakes and breakfast cereals and bars. They have three significant properties:

1. Added sucrose (table sugar) or fructose, which is the sweet part of table sugar. Think muffins and cakes.
2. Many of the carbs already exist as single or double sugar units, saving our gut the need to do any enzyme work at all! These are absorbed super-fast, causing a spike in our blood glucose (sugar).
3. Fructose puts the liver under strain to convert it to glucose or triglycerides (fats) that are stored in the liver. Excess fructose causes peripheral obesity and fatty liver disease.

Worth noting is the *baguette de tradition française*, which by French law may only have four ingredients: flour, water, yeast and common salt. By contrast, most bread in the Western Pattern Diet contains so much added sugar, it is really cake! In a 2020 judgment, an Irish court ruled that the bread served by the Subway chain across some 110 countries could not in fact be defined as bread because of its high sugar content.[1]

CLASSIFYING CARBOHYDRATES

Confusion occurs because different terminology has been used over the years. We will stick with this simple classification.

1. Quickly digested (refined and super-refined carbohydrates with little or no fibre) = Bad.
2. Slowly digested (unrefined carbohydrates with a high fibre/roughage content) = Good.

We saw above how quickly digested carbs have little to no fibre and are broken down easily by our gut enzymes into sugars, crossing into our blood quickly.

When we eat these, they raise our blood glucose rapidly and significantly. In the first revolution we got *refined carbohydrates*, and in the second we got *super-refined carbohydrates*.

Slowly digested carbs, also known as *unrefined carbohydrates*, are naturally occurring and high in cellulose fibre. When we eat them, they cause a slower and lower rise in blood glucose (Figure 4.3). Examples are whole fruits, beans, lentils, potato skins, cabbage, carrots, Brussels sprouts, broccoli and so on. In other words, proper whole vegetables.[2]

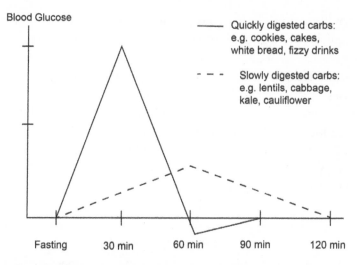

Figure 4.3. Blood glucose after quickly and slowly digested carbohydrates.

CARBOHYDRATE FIBRE: THE GEM OF NUTRITIONAL HEALTH

Please, please, please know that fibre is a diamond, a true gem of our nutritional health. Fibre has lots of cellulose chains with bonds that our digestive enzymes cannot break down. It is also known as roughage and there are two types:

- Solid fibre is non-water soluble and acts like a mini scaffold in the gut. Any carbs that are waiting to be digested are surrounded by this scaffold, making its digestion and absorption into the blood more difficult. It increases the speed at which food travels through the gut, again reducing its absorption, or bioavailability. It is undigested, feeds the gut bugs and forms a bulky stool, reducing our risk of colon cancer and diverticulosis. It also surrounds the food with liquid fibre.
- Liquid fibre is a water-soluble gel that also surrounds the food, making it even harder for the food to be digested and absorbed from the small intestine into our blood. This helps to pass the food down to the large gut, where it is digested and fermented by our gut bugs, which keeps them healthy and helps to increase the good ones and their overall diversity. This is crucial for the health of the gut itself as well as mental and physical health and weight loss (see Chapter 7).

Dietary fibre draws in water and bulks up our stool, making it move more quickly though the large bowel and helping to produce a stool that is readily passed. It reduces blood glucose, blood insulin, constipation and reduces the so-called 'bad' type of blood cholesterol. Fibre increases large gut fermentation, whereby our friendly gut bugs produce good chemicals that make us happy, and gas, which becomes good healthy farts. If you're not farting, ask yourself if you are getting that 30 g of fibre a day. If you want a takeaway message as important as any, it would be: MORE FIBRE, SOME STARCH, LITTLE SUGAR, NO FRUCTOSE.

DON'T JUICE FRUIT

In 2020 the world produced some 2 million tonnes of frozen concentrated orange juice (FCOJ). Since 1950 it has been keenly traded on commodity futures' markets. It is a worldwide favourite breakfast staple. Fruit juices have no solid fibre or liquid fibre; it has been bashed out of them in the processing. They are associated with insulin resistance, weight gain, liver and pancreatic stress and metabolic syndrome. Fruit juices contain the sugars glucose and fructose in roughly equal amounts, except when extra fructose is added in the form of high fructose corn syrup (HFCS). Fructose stresses the liver, and in the US excessive consumption of fructose is now the major cause of non-alcoholic fatty liver disease or NAFLD, present in over 25 per cent of US adults.[3] Fruits are designed to be eaten whole, so their fibre slows absorption, allowing much of the glucose and fructose to pass to the large bowel, feeding your gut bugs, rather than you.

There are no fruit juices in our fridge, not at home, not at Whisperer HQ!

BIOAVAILABILITY, GLYCAEMIC INDEX (GI) AND GLYCAEMIC LOAD (GL)

Bioavailability is a simple concept. Imagine a drug smuggler who has swallowed 50 condoms, all containing class A drugs. If one condom bursts, the smuggler will die, because the drug becomes 'bioavailable' – passes from the gut, across the gut wall and into the bloodstream, resulting in a fatal overdose. So the drug smuggler is hoping, and possibly praying, for zero bioavailability. That is, hoping the class As pass out with the stool, completely unchanged.

The glycaemic index (GI) of a food is how quickly it raises blood glucose. In other words, how quickly it is digested and absorbed into the blood. GI is scored as low being below 55, medium from 56 to 69, and high being above 70. Unsurprisingly, eating raw sugar has the reference value of 100.

LOW GI < 55		MEDIUM 56—69		HIGH >70	
Steel-cut porridge oats	51	Pineapple	66	Glucose	100
Banana (not juiced)	50	Couscous	65	Cornflakes	85
Apple (not juiced)	46	Sweet potatoes	59	Instant porridge	79
Milk 'full-fat'	40	Wild rice	57	White bread	77
Orange (not juiced)	36	Rolled porridge	56	Brown bread	73
Lentils	32			Boiled rice	73
Beans	28			Chips/fries	70
Broccoli	15			Orange juice	65
Lettuce	15				
Tomatoes	15				
Full-fat yoghurt	14				

Figure 4.4. High, medium and low GI carbohydrates.

The concept is simple: give a subject 50 grams of a particular carbohydrate, then chart the blood glucose over time. When you do that for refined carbohydrates you get a frightening chart like the one overleaf (Figure 4.5).

The glycaemic load (GL) takes into account real food in the real world. It takes a portion of that food and looks at the carbohydrate content. It then combines this with the GI of that carbohydrate and expresses this as a number. Low GL is 10 or less, moderate is 11–19 and high is 20 and above. For example, a watermelon and a doughnut have similar GI at a very high 76, but when we look at how much of this glucose there is per portion, we see that the doughnut is still very high at a GL of 17, but the slice of watermelon is around 3, very low. So, you now have an idea of what your blood glucose will be doing per real-life portion of each food. In real life bioavailability and GL change with cooking methods and other foodstuffs consumed. Carbohydrate absorption is reduced when combined with fats, proteins or fibre, as we have seen.

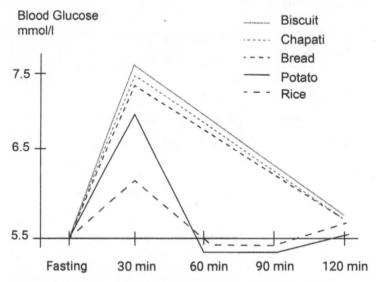

Figure 4.5. Blood glucose afer eating a variety of refined and super-refined carbohydrates. (Graph adapted from reference 2).

BIOVAILABILITY AND MICRONUTRIENTS

Our ability to absorb micronutrients is dependent on our genes, our environment and the constituents of our microbiome. We are very individual, and so is the bioavailability of micronutrients. The packet may say 100 per cent of our recommended daily intake (RDI) for iron, selenium or zinc, but it doesn't stop there; the question is how much will you absorb? If you don't absorb it, your body can't use it. And the answer is complex because it varies between individuals.

BLOOD GLUCOSE LEVELS

To keep us safe, our hormones maintain our blood glucose within a critical range. To confuse us all, the units of measurement have changed in the last decade, so I'll use both. The first figure is mmol/L and the second mg/dL.

The normal range for our blood sugar before a meal is 4.00–5.40 mmol/L (72–99). Two hours after a meal it is up to 7.8 mmol/L (140). The importance of having this normal range cannot be overstated and our hormones maintain it with great alacrity. When we wake in the morning our hormones adjust our blood sugar upwards, so we arise bright and cheerful.

Low blood glucose

Hypo is short for hypoglycaemia, a term for blood glucose falling below the normal range. Hypos can cause unconsciousness and if severe may result in death. Hypos usually occur in people with known type 1 diabetes (on insulin), as a result of either over-treatment or too little food. When people with type 2 diabetes (on tablets) lose weight, they can suffer hypos, so medical supervision of medication reduction is required.

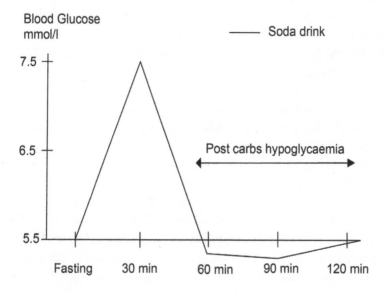

Figure 4.6. High blood glucose falling to suboptimal (hypo) after high GI carbs, refined or super-refined.

The symptoms are similar to carb-hunger: shakes, tingling lips, pallor, dizziness, fainting, irregular heartbeat, irritability, depression, anxiety and mood swings. To a lesser extent this happens in healthy people after eating or drinking super-refined carbs; you can see on the graph that there is a period of lowish blood glucose after an hour or two (Figure 4.6). In my medical school days, I would enjoy my Big Mac, large fries, ketchup and large Coke, only to feel very sleepy two hours later. It took me decades to find out why!

High blood glucose

This is very important. At the Diet Whisperer we call this well-trodden journey 'The Metabolic Bus': a diet rich in refined and super-refined carbs, then insulin resistance, then obesity, then high fasting insulin, then high blood glucose, then metabolic syndrome and then a whole host of conditions along with type 2 diabetes (Figure 1.1).

High blood sugar levels are associated with very nasty inflammatory and atherogenic (furring up) changes in blood vessels all over the body, known as cardiovascular disease or CVD. This is associated not only with heart attacks and strokes, but with kidney failure, infection and lower limb amputation. In the first two decades after diagnosis of diabetes, more than half of all sufferers have eye disease. So, high blood sugar is not to be sniffed at.

The biggest risk factor for all these complications is *length of time*, with the stopwatch starting when the insulin levels rise and insulin resistance is present.

But there is really, really, REALLY great news. For the majority of people, insulin resistance can be reversed simply by following the whisperer plan. The further down the road you have gone, and the larger the number of metabolic syndrome components you have (see Chapter 8), the longer the reversal process will be. We've seen many whisperers with type 2 diabetes go into full remission. For some the diabetes will persist, but it will be much better controlled, tablets reduced, obesity gone and complications less severe. As you steadily improve your knowledge you will gain the skills to take back control of your metabolic changes, including insulin resistance, blood glucose, your weight, and your health.

ARTIFICIAL SWEETENERS

Note that all zero-calorie drinks have the sugar replaced with artificial sweeteners. There is growing evidence that these are just as bad, but for other reasons. They may adversely affect the delicate balances in our gut microbiome. They are known to be associated with cardiovascular disease, strokes and obesity. And they are highly addictive. So, sorry, they screw you up too.

READ THE LABEL

Firstly, if it's got a label, it's not food. But, if you wish to eat this stuff, read the label. Big Food corporates use so many names to disguise the sugar that they add to products to get you hooked. Buyer beware. The names of sugar include, but are far from limited to:

Agave nectar, Barley malt, Beet sugar, Blackstrap molasses, Brown rice syrup, Brown sugar, Buttered syrup, Cane juice crystals, Cane sugar, Caramel, Carob syrup, Caster sugar, Coconut sugar, Corn syrup, Corn syrup solids, Crystalline fructose, Date sugar, Demerara sugar, D-ribose Galactose, Dextrin, Dextrose, Diastatic, Evaporated cane juice, Florida crystals, Fructose, Fruit juice, Fruit juice concentrate, Glucose, Glucose solids, Golden sugar, Golden syrup, Grape sugar, HFCS (high fructose corn syrup), Honey icing sugar, Lactose, Malt ethyl, Maltol, Malt syrup, Maltodextrin, Maltose, Maple syrup molasses, Muscovado sugar, Panela sugar, Raw sugar, Refiner's syrup, Rice syrup, Sorghum syrup, Sucanat, Sucrose (table sugar), Treacle sugar, Turbinado sugar, Yellow sugar.

FRUCTOSE: ANOTHER LIVER TOXIN?

The fructose in high fructose corn syrup (HFCS) is indicated by its suffix number. So HFCS55 is 55 per cent fructose and 45 per cent glucose. HFCS45 is used in foodstuffs like breakfast cereals and HFCS55 is used in soft drinks like the fizzy drinks we talked about earlier. Glucose, when consumed slowly and in moderate amounts, is burned and any excess converted into muscle or liver glycogen. The real problem with fructose is that it causes so many health problems. Excess fructose is converted into fats in the liver, damages glucose metabolism, causes insulin resistance, and increases the ageing process through the Maillard process. It also damages liver mitochondria. It causes non-alcoholic fatty liver disease and increases hunger by directly causing leptin resistance. You have been warned: avoid it (Figure 4.7).[3,4]

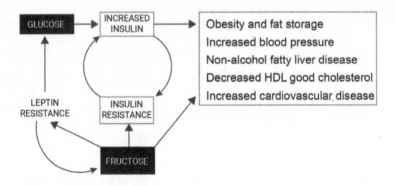

Figure 4.7. The effects of dietary fructose and glucose on insulin resistance and health. Note the direct effects of fructose.[4]

GLUCOSE, METABOLIC STRESS AND OBESITY

We can see from the chart in Figure 4.8 that the type of carbohydrate eaten changes the metabolic stress and obesity. To think through this, we need to understand the different carbs. Firstly, natural foods high in cellulose fibre, like greens, protect us from metabolic stress and insulin resistance and help us to lose weight. These should be the biggest portion on our plate; they are our microbiome protectors. Then whole foods like potato skins, which are low in glucose, high in nutrients and high in the good carbs, or cellulose fibre. Then we move on to naturally occurring starches, like potatoes and rice. Next up are the refined starches, made from flour, like pasta and the *baguette de tradition française*. These contain flour and natural starches; the carb chains are glucose-glucose-glucose. Next come the chains made of a glucose-fructose mix, when table sugar, HFCS or other sugars are added; these are found in foods like cakes, sweets and fizzy drinks. The exception here is berries and fruit; great foods because eaten whole they contain fibre and would be between 1 and 2 on the chart. But juice the fibre out of them and they go straight to number 10, with 100 per cent maximum obesogenic stress. Also very high up are any foods with added sugar or HFCS. This causes all the problems listed above, and even our bread and burger buns are riddled with the stuff.

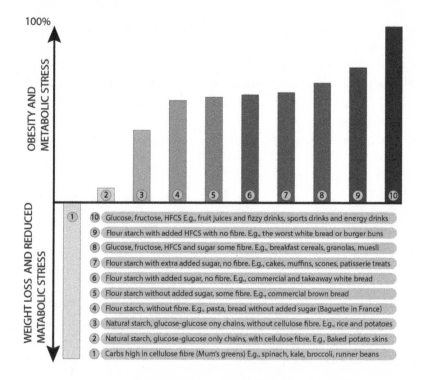

The chart shows a vertical axis labeled "OBESITY AND METABOLIC STRESS" (top, to 100%) and "WEIGHT LOSS AND REDUCED MATABOLIC STRESS" (bottom). Bars numbered 2 through 10.

10 — Glucose, fructose, HFCS E.g., fruit juices and fizzy drinks, sports drinks and energy drinks

9 — Flour starch with added HFCS with no fibre. E.g., the worst white bread or burger buns

8 — Glucose, fructose, HFCS and sugar some fibre. E.g., breakfast cereals, granolas, muesli

7 — Flour starch with extra added sugar, no fibre. E.g., cakes, muffins, scones, patisserie treats

6 — Flour starch with added sugar, no fibre. E.g., commercial and takeaway white bread

5 — Flour starch without added sugar, some fibre. E.g., commercial brown bread

4 — Flour starch, without fibre. E.g., pasta, bread without added sugar (Baguette in France)

3 — Natural starch, glucose-glucose ony chains, without cellulose fibre. E.g., rice and potatoes

2 — Natural starch, glucose-glucose only chains, with cellulose fibre. E.g., Baked potato skins

1 — Carbs high in cellulose fibre (Mum's greens) E.g., spinach, kale, broccoli, runner beans

CHAPTER WHISPERINGS

- Increase your fibre to over 30 g a day.
- Avoid all fruit juices and breakfast cereals, particularly those with HFCS.
- Carbohydrates are stored in our body as long chains called glycogen.
- Carbohydrates are stored in plants as long chains called starch which we can digest, or cellulose which we cannot.
- Carbohydrates after absorption can be burned, or stored as glycogen and fat.
- Slowly digested unrefined carbohydrates, or fibre, are essential for our gut bugs' health.
- Carbohydrates come in two types; quickly digested (high GI; refined and super-refined=bad) and slowly digested (low GI; unrefined; fibre=good).
- Refined and super-refined carbohydrates have increased 50-fold in our diets over the past 100 years.
- The glycaemic index (GI) of carbohydrates indicates their ability to raise blood glucose.

- The glycaemic load (GL) of food indicates the blood glucose 'per portion' of that food.
- The body's hormones maintain a base level of glucose in our blood.
- High consumption of refined and super-refined high GI carbohydrates leads to raised insulin, insulin resistance, metabolic syndrome and diabetes.
- Insulin resistance is the beginning of our journey on the metabolic bus.

5

FATS

A misconception remains a misconception, even when it is shared by the majority of people.

Leo Tolstoy

FAT STORES

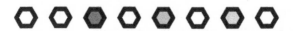

FATS ARE ALSO LINKED IN CHAINS

FATS

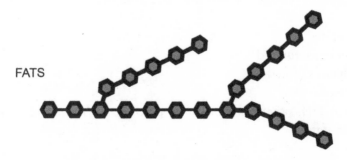

STORED FATS LINKED = TRIGLYCERIDE

Figure 5.1. Fats are chains, broken down for digestion and absorbed into our lymph and blood. They are stored as new chains, with branches in our fat stores.

FAT MYTHS AND FACTS

Let's get three facts right out there straight away; facts that are worth repeating until you are relieved of your own misconceptions about fat:

1. Saturated fats make you *neither fat, nor ill.*
2. Low-fat foods *do not make you lose weight.*
3. High-fat foods *make you healthy and lose weight.*

Low-fat foods make you fat because perfectly healthy and essential fats have been replaced with super-refined carbohydrates. Fats are great foods and fats do not make you ill; refined carbohydrates make you ill, and super-refined carbohydrates make you *iller!*

Feel free to read that sentence as often as you like. Many years ago, when I first came across this fact, it made me quite angry. In fact, I'm still quite peeved writing it. We have been fed this 'fat is bad' drivel for over 40 years. And it's just plain wrong.

Fats are our major energy storage macronutrient, and like carbohydrates are comprised of long chains of fats, linked together (Figure 5.1). Like carbs, they are taken from our bloodstream after eating, then stored in fat cells at the behest of the hormone insulin (see Chapter 10). Fat is our friend and a great macronutrient, as you'll discover. The exception to the rule is the man-made trans fats; they are absolute killers and should be avoided at all costs. Trans fats are banned in most countries in the world. Pathetically, the UK has a voluntary code, which for scurrilous owners of restaurants and takeaways means no code at all; they can continue to be peddled, within the law.

We classify our dietary fats into five groups:

1. Saturated
2. Monounsaturated
3. Polyunsaturated
4. Cholesterol
5. Trans fats, otherwise known as partially hydrogenated fats, or killer fats!

For the scientifically inquisitive, the chains of saturated fats have no double bonds, while monounsaturated chains have one, and polyunsaturated more than one.

SATURATED FATS (SF)

These have been vilified for the past 50 years. They were reduced in the Western diet at the behest of the US Department of Agriculture Food and Nutrition Service (USDA-FNS) and quickly followed by the UK. These are the fats found in meat, dairy, whole milk and butter, cheese, dark chicken meat, chicken breast skin, lard and oils such as coconut and palm. The original data used to create these regulations has been reanalysed and we now know that the conclusions were just plain wrong. By cutting them out and replacing them with refined carbohydrates, we have started to see more cancer, heart disease, obesity and chronic diseases. These fats are a great part of a healthy diet, and do not cause heart disease. It is processed foods and refined and super-refined carbs that do that.[1,2] Scientists continue to debate this matter on both sides, even today!

MONOUNSATURATED FATTY ACIDS (MUFAs)

There are 13 of these found in the human diet, with oleic acid comprising about 90 per cent. Most extra virgin olive oils have 85 per cent MUFAs. Extra virgin olive oil (EVOO) is made from the cold-pressed juice from olives, without heating. There is a mass of evidence for the health benefits of MUFAs, particularly when replacing dietary saturated fat and refined carbohydrates with them. Benefits include reduced blood pressure, lowered bad cholesterol and increased vitamin E levels. High oleic acid has been linked with reduced insulin resistance in normal subjects and people with diabetes. Observational studies have found reductions in breast cancer risk. People on the Mediterranean diet, which is rich in MUFAs, have shown reduced 'bad' cholesterol. MUFAs are also associated with reduced inflammatory markers, implicated in so many chronic illnesses, from cancer and arthritis to cardiovascular disease and ageing. They also reduce inflammation within fat cells.[3,4,5]

POLYUNSATURATED FATTY ACIDS (PUFAs)

Since I gave my first lecture in Switzerland on this subject in 2010, it has been a source of fascination for me, revealing some real health gems. Firstly, the terminology; there are three types of PUFAs: omega-9s, omega-6s and omega-3s. Omega-9s, which are mainly oleic acid have been discussed above under MUFAs.

Some facts about PUFAs:

- Omega-3 and omega-6 are 'essential' dietary fats; our body cannot make them.
- Both omega-3 and omega-6 are essential for our overall health.
- Omega-6s are pro-inflammatory.
- Omega-3s are anti-inflammatory.
- When you take non-steroidal 'anti-inflammatory' drugs, they work to block the omega-6 pathways in your body.

- Omega-6s and omega-3s compete for the same enzyme to be activated.
- The importance lies in the ratio, or balance between them in our weekly food; what we call the omega-6 to omega-3 ratio; or 6/3 ratio.
- A blood test can measure the 6/3 ratio in red blood cell membranes.

We know the majority of modern illnesses have an inflammatory component. Common sense points us to the obvious question: what was the omega-6/-3 ratio 100 years ago, and what is it now? The shocking answer to this question is this:

In our distant ancestors, the ratio was 1/1; in our relatives just 100 years ago it was 2.5/1; and now in the worst Western Pattern Diet the 6/3 ratio is 50/1. That means for every anti-inflammatory omega-3 in our diet, we have 50 pro-inflammatory omega-6s. That is a staggering figure. It means our bodies are crammed full of inflammation-producing omega-6s.

So, in the last century, harmful super-refined carbs have increased 100-fold, and the pro-inflammatory omega-6/-3 ratio 20-fold. But with just a little understanding, you can positively change your health by altering these ratios in your favour. Both for you and your loved ones. And that is a life-changer. Get those two factors right and you really will be a new and improved YOU.

This high omega-6 to omega-3 ratio is associated with:[6,7,8,9,10,11]

- Increased asthma: reducing the ratio to 5/1 improves asthma; increasing to 10/1 makes it worse.
- Increased arthritis inflammation.
- Dry eyes.
- Increased cancer risks.
- Increased mortality in breast cancer.
- Increased cardiovascular disease at ratios over 4/1.
- Increased platelet aggregation, making blood sticky and prone to clotting.
- Increased inflammation in chronic renal disease.
- Increased inflammation in sepsis.
- Increased inflammation in acute pancreatitis.
- Increased inflammation in peripheral vascular disease.

- Increased inflammatory bowel disease.
- Increased autoimmune disease.
- Increased insulin resistance.
- Increased metabolic syndrome and type 2 diabetes.
- Increased obesity.
- Increased chronic inflammatory diseases.
- Increased vaginal inflammatory conditions.

A high 6/3 ratio combined with quickly digested carbs proves to be very damaging. This list gets the message over loud and clear – and it is far from exhaustive. So, the science backs up the logic that we should rebalance our ratios as low as we can, and to aim for an omega-6/-3 ratio of 4/1 or below.

Names of PUFAs
Omega-3s are ALA, EPA and DHA (alpha-linoleic acid; eicosapentaenoic acid and docosahexaenoic acid). In the body ALA can be converted into EPA and then DHA, so is technically the only essential PUFA. However, as less then 20 per cent is converted, consuming EPA and DHA in food is necessary to increase levels. Omega-6s are linoleic acid and arachidonic acid.

Sources of Omega-3s
Oily fish and cod liver oil are the best sources. Mackerel, salmon, herring, sardines and anchovies are the richest sources.

For vegetarians there are algae sources for omega-3s such as chlorella and spirulina, which have many other minerals and vitamins to boot. Their mineral and vitamin contents are quite different from animal sources, so taking both is an option. Research has shown them to have some benefits in reducing triglycerides, LDL (bad) cholesterol and blood pressure. They also contain lutein and zeaxanthin, good for eye health and used to reduce the progression of macular degeneration. They have been shown to increase insulin sensitivity and have antioxidant properties. They have been used as foodstuffs around the world for hundreds of years.

Sources of Omega-6s

Safflower oil, sunflower oil, corn oil and soybean oil are the major sources in our diet, so we need to really watch our frying habits to limit the omega-6s. Omega-6s are also found in corn, some nuts and meat. In meat, omega-6s are increased by the process of fattening involving grains. Grass-feeding naturally increases omega-3s.

Omega-6s and omega-3s are often both present in foods. So, to be clear in what we want to achieve we need to look at the ratios. Our ratios should be less than 4/1 (omega-6/-3). Men need to limit omega-6s to under 17 grams a day. Men also need over 4 grams of omega-3s to hit the ideal ratio. Daily figures for women are under 12 grams of omega-6s and over 3 grams of omega-3s.

Eating good healthy foods is always good advice. When we eat grass-fed beef, we get a much healthier omega-6/-3 ratio. In fact, the difference is due to more omega-3s rather than fewer omega-6s, which is consistent with current science. The ratio changes from 7/1 to 3/1. Fantastic for all the reasons stated above. The same applies to other meat such as lamb and venison. But a word of warning: the terminology you want is not only 'grass-fed', but also 'grass-finished'. The taste and good health benefits of the 3/1 ratio are lost if the cattle are fed grain (often in farming called nuts) at the end to fatten them up. So, be specific, and if your butcher doesn't understand you, find a new butcher!

The tables (Figure 5.2 and Figure 5.3) give you an idea of the foods that cause our 6/3 ratios to be healthy or unhealthy. It is worth noting that extra virgin olive oil (EVOO) has mainly MUFAs and that 15 per cent of PUFAs are in a ratio of 10/1. In spite of this, EVOO is by far the healthiest oil. Also note how the ratios change dramatically from extremely good to extremely bad in canned fish depending on whether they are canned in vegetable oil or water. And when you look at the figures for commonly used vegetable cooking oils, you realise that foods like chips, crisps and deep-fried poppadums are cooked in vegetable oils rich in omega-6s. So although delicious, they are simply a vehicle for transferring inflammatory omega-6s into your body. Like a bus crammed with omega-6s, heading your way. Ugh.

The greatest health benefits come from the magic triad of regular exercise, good diet and not smoking. Get all three right and your risk of heart disease goes down by a staggering 80 per cent. So, like everything, doing one thing will only have a small effect on its own. We know that people who follow this magic triad and supplement with vitamin D and omega-3s get *marginal b*enefits from the supplements. But in more vulnerable people like the obese, people with kidney disease or people with low-fish diets, taking vitamin D and omega-3s can reduce risks of heart disease significantly.[12,13]

Food (100 mg)	Omega-6 (mg)	Omega-3 (mg)	Ratio
Sea salmon	170	2000	1:12
Herring	250	2500	1:10
Tinned tuna (in water)	9	270	1:30
Tinned tuna (in sunflower oil)	2680	200	13:1
Crab	80	480	1:60
Cod	80	480	1:60

Figure 5.2. The ratio of inflammatory omega-6s to anti-inflammatory omega-3s in healthy foods. Note when water (brine) is replaced by sunflower oil in tuna, the ratio goes from very good to very bad.

Oil	Omega-6 %	Omega-3 %
Sunflower or safflower oil	70	0
Corn oil	55	0
Peanut oil	30	0
Soybean oil	51	7
Canola oil	20	9
Walnut oil	52	10

Figure 5.3. Adverse ratio of omega-6 to omega-3 in cooking oils. Soybean oils form up to 10% of the modern US diet.

CHOLESTEROL

Firstly, cholesterol. The bad boy, right? Wrong. To make it water-soluble, cholesterol is transported in our blood by lipoproteins, a combination of fat and protein. Hence the suffix -C (see below). Cholesterol is required in the human body by every cell membrane, in cellular functionality, and to make hormones like oestrogen and testosterone, as well as our fight or flight hormone, cortisol. It plays a major role in the structure of our myelin, the protective sheath around our nerves, allowing them to functional normally. It is quite simply a vital part of human life. The lipoproteins are classified by weight.

The so-called bad boy

The low-density lipoprotein LDL, or cholesterol level LDL-C, has had the most bad press because of its role in atherosclerosis: the furring up of our arteries. Atherosclerosis in turn leads to strokes, heart attacks and early death. However, LDL-C *must* be further classified by size, with the particle LDL-Ps being the smallest and greatest implicated. The atherogenic furring of arteries is highly associated with LDL-P and another lipoprotein called Apolipoprotein B or ApoB. These help to explain why 30 per cent of heart attacks occur in people with low or normal LDL-C. The larger LDL-P particles are thought to be protective, so we must determine which type of LDL-C we have. When you get your cholesterol tested, you must request your LDL particle levels (LDL-P), as these are correlated with a tripling of cardiovascular risk. High triglycerides (TGs) correlate with high LDL-P and vice versa. In the over-sixties a raised *total* LDL-C correlates with better immunity, and reduced deaths from all causes.[14]

The so-called good boy

High-density lipoprotein (HDL) hoovers up cholesterol around the body and returns it to the liver for processing. And HDL-C is known to be protective for our arteries.

So, now you know which cholesterol tests you need and why. If you want further information, go to the website, where we keep the current best tests and interpretation of results. With cholesterol, one thing is for sure: there is no scientific consensus. This is far from sorted, so watch this space! And *A Statin Free Life* by Aseem Malhotra and *Fat Chance* by Robert Lustig are good starting points; see Further Reading.

Dietary cholesterol only increases LDL cholesterol in so called 'hyper-responders' and in these people it tends to be the larger, less dangerous form. In the same people it also increases the protective HDL, so the ratio of good to bad remains stable. Egg yolks, particularly rich in cholesterol, are associated neither with increased heart disease nor raised LDL cholesterol. When our bodies digest cholesterol, liver cholesterol production goes down, and when we eat less our liver churns out more from the stores. Cholesterol rich foods are healthy, delicious and highly nutritious, and include avocados, nuts, eggs, liver, shellfish, oily fish (salmon, mackerel, sardines) and *grass-finished* meat like beef, lamb and venison.

I hate to see friends ruining their lives, miserable on low-fat diets and statins from their doctors. The controversy concerning statins is beyond the scope of this book, but suffice it to say, not in our house! If you are a normal healthy adult and want to reduce your cholesterol, which in old money means lower your 'bad' LDL and increase your 'good' HDL, there are very easy ways that are misery-free. Firstly, get the right blood tests. Then follow my top ten tips to reduce bad cholesterol.

1. Exercise (if you've been sedentary, walking for 30 minutes a day will do).
2. Reduce insulin resistance.
3. Reduce weight.
4. Don't smoke.
5. Reduce your vegetable oils that are high in omega-6s and increase your omega-3s.
6. Increase dietary fibre.
7. Increase you MUFAs, as per the Mediterranean diet.
8. Eat plant sterols, but not in margarine spreads that contain trans fats (read the label and see below).
9. Eat a minimum of two portions of oily fish per week.
10. If you don't eat fish, take fish oil daily – 1000 mg or 1 gram of fish oil contains 300 mg of EPA and DHA combined. And the daily recommended intakes for EPA and DHA are 1600 mg for men and 1100 mg for women. So, 4–5 grams of fish oil for men and 3–4 grams for women.

All this is part of the *whisperer lifestyle*. Enjoy your steak, cooked on a cast-iron skillet, dressed with butter, with a lovely plate of buttered greens and mushrooms. If you must have chips, cook them in goose or beef fat, as a delicious *treat meal*.

KILLER TRANS FATS

Trans fats are also known as partially hydrogenated fats. This is crucial information because these are the very bad boys, and there is nothing *so-called* about it. There is full consensus among the scientists. They are commonly found in spreads, biscuits and margarine. They are irrefutably linked to obesity, cancer, immune diseases, neuro-degenerative diseases and cardiovascular disease. They are banned in wise countries like Canada, Denmark, Austria and more recently the USA. There is still widespread use in UK restaurants and takeaways. If you use one regularly, ask them to show you the packaging and photograph it. Do your own research and see if it contains partially hydrogenated oils (trans fats).

It is the WHO intention that all trans fats be eradicated from the human diet by 2023.

In my cooking:
- Fried eggs: gently on a slow low heat with EVOO.
- Casseroles: low heat (175°C) and long EVOO (below its smoke point of 195°C.)
- Thick chips: beef dripping, or goose fat, and a rare treat.
- Stir fries: walnut oil.
- Banned in our house: corn oil, sunflower, safflower and canola (rapeseed) oils.
- Never trans fats, from any source; *run away quickly.*
- Reused trans fats, almost the scariest of them all; *run away, but even more quickly.*
- In China, there is a trade in sewer oil, which is vegetable oil extracted from the sewers; *I simply have no comment.*

KEYS VERSUS YUDKIN. THE WINNERS WERE CORPORATE FOOD. THE LOSERS WERE US

In 1970s America, the greatest controversy of all was Ancel Keys convincing the American people that a low-fat diet was the right way. In the UK John Yudkin was telling us that too much sugar was the problem. After much debate, the argument was won by Keys.

Keys was the first person to propose that saturated animal fat was correlated with heart disease. In the 1960s, heart disease was a new problem and of increasing concern to governments in the West, and particularly in the US. Keys embarked on the Seven Countries Study, presenting correlations between intake of animal saturated fats and 'reported' (and that's an important word) blood vessel atheromatous heart disease at death.

There was much criticism of Keys's study, in particular over correlation versus causation and the fact that he reduced the study from his original hypothesis of twenty countries to seven. One of the countries he left out was France, where saturated fats are enjoyed and which has the world's second-to-bottom heart disease scores. Put simply, at best this is not good science.

THE IMPACT OF KEYS'S WORK

The day that Ancel Keys persuaded the politicians running the US Senate committee on diet and nutrition that food must contain less fat, the world fell into perilous times. And it was really easy to get the corporates and farmers on board because:

- it would be a revolution in the food industry and
- America's farming belt was now producing millions of acres of corn, from which the sugar substitute high fructose corn syrup is cheaply produced as a by-product.

The food corporates and their food scientists went to work removing the fat from everything we eat. The world of 'low-fat' food was born. But the biggest hurdle lay ahead.

LOW FAT YOGHURT AND THE RISE OF HFCS

When the fat was taken out, the yoghurt tasted bad. So bad, it tasted like wallpaper paste, with the wallpaper paste removed. Back to the drawing board.

Eureka! Why not replace the fat with sugar? The taste was great, but the maths didn't work. And so it was substituted for ultra-sweet high fructose corn syrup. Cheap as chips – and a form of human poison, now in everything from yoghurts to cereal and fizzy drinks.

Food company owners, scientists and managers may have entered corporate nirvana, but the rest of us were about to lose control of our hormones. We were blindfolded and herded onto the metabolic bus that would pass the stops of insulin resistance, obesity, metabolic syndrome, diabetes, cardiovascular disease and cancer, en route to an early demise. But right now it's your time to take your chance. Your time to alight that bus, and run!

CHAPTER WHISPERINGS

- Low-fat foods have the fat replaced with sugar or HFCS.
- Low-fat foods make you fat, and ill.
- Saturated fats are part of a healthy balanced diet and important in weight loss
- PUFA omega-6s are pro-inflammatory and are associated with many health problems.
- PUFA omega-3s are anti-inflammatory and associated with better health.
- Modern diets have omega-6/-3 ratios up to 50/1, when it should be under 4/1.
- Vegetable cooking oils are crammed with omega-6s.
- Oily fish is crammed with great omega-3s.
- MUFAs are a big part of the Mediterranean diet: EVOO, olives, avocados.
- Any cholesterol blood tests should assess your small particle LDL-Ps.
- Blood cholesterol is 80 per cent produced in the liver, 20 per cent in the diet.
- Bad cholesterol comes from a bad liver, damaged by high sugar diets and fructose.
- There are ten simple ways to reduce your cholesterol.
- Check for partially hydrogenated trans fats in your food, particularly in restaurants and takeaways you frequently use. Pop in when it's quiet and ask them. If they won't show you what they cook with, move on.
- UK and US government advice to reduce saturated fat is wrong and 40 years out of date.

6

PROTEINS

The doctors of the future will no longer treat the human
frame with drugs, but rather will cure and prevent
disease with nutrition.

Thomas Edison

AMINO ACIDS x 21

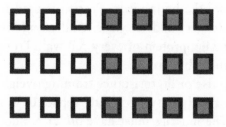

INDIVIDUAL ESSENTIAL (9) AND NON-ESSENTIAL (12)

PROTEIN

AMINO ACIDS LINKED = POLYPEPTIDE

Figure 6.1. Proteins are made up from a mixture of amino acids, both essential and
non-essential. These are broken down during digestion ready for absorption into the
blood. From here they are remade into new chains forming new proteins in the body.

Our third macronutrient needs little introduction and is truly ubiquitous. In modern parlance, it is 'literally' found in every part of the human body. *Protos*, from the Greek for 'first'. Like our other macronutrients, protein is eaten as a long chain of pearls, broken down in digestion so the individual pearls can be absorbed (Figure 6.1). This time the pearls are not sugars, nor fats, but amino acids, the building blocks of protein. We can see from the diagram that there are 21 amino acids, of which 9 are essential, meaning they cannot be manufactured by our body. When we string them together, they become polypeptides and when they get even longer, we get proteins. Protein is what makes up our bones, muscles, tendons and ligaments. It allows us our movement and gives us our strength. It also gives our bodies the collagen that supports our tissues and skin. Collagen decreases with ageing; a process speeded up by a quickly digested carb diet and slowed by fasting.

There is so much more to protein than the muscles we immediately think of. It is required for hormones, skin, nails and hair, and haemoglobin. We have carrier proteins that transport lactic acid out of our burning muscles during endurance events. Ferritin is a protein that stores and releases the body's iron. Protein is used for making antibodies, cell messengers and enzymes. And along with fats, it is of course part of the lipoprotein of every cell wall. Protein in our beautiful bodies is truly ubiquitous.

When we exercise or do resistance training (weights) our muscles become damaged and are subsequently repaired over the next three to seven days. The muscles must have *all* 21 amino acids available for those repairs to take place. And there is the 'steal effect' – if you exercise your arms (say) and you don't have enough dietary protein, your body will steal it from your legs. And vice versa; protein will always be pinched from somewhere else if your diet is deficient.

Lean meat, being muscle, is mainly protein. Beef for example is 65 per cent water, 25 per cent protein and 10 per cent fat. No carbs. It also contains many micronutrients such as selenium, iron, zinc, cholesterol and vitamins B3, B6 and B12. As well as dairy, there are many vegetable sources of protein too; tofu, lentils, chickpeas, spirulina and chlorella are all rich sources.

SARCOPENIA AND METABOLISM

If sarcopenia is a new word to you, this could be life-changing. Our muscles are known as lean tissue. After the age of 35 we lose muscle every year for the rest of our life (Figure 6.2). This happens to everyone and this is sarcopenia. We lose between 3 and 8 per cent of our lean tissue weight per decade over the age of 35.

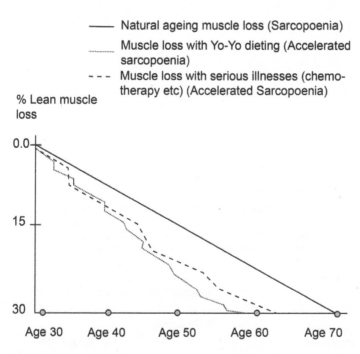

Figure 6.2 . Natural vs accelerated sarcopenia (muscle loss) after age 30 in percentage terms.

Although this happens naturally with ageing, it is accelerated by yo-yo dieting; the repeated cycles of diet, lose weight (muscle and fat) and then put it back on again (fat). You will see from the chart that accelerated sarcopenia occurs in serious illnesses and shows a similar pattern to repeated dieting (Figure 6.3 and Figure 6.4). So diets are a cause of accelerated sarcopenia. This matters a lot, as a lack of muscle is associated with falls in the elderly[1] and, in the very elderly, falls have the same prognosis as a diagnosis of cancer. So the message is very simple: build up your balance, strength and muscles throughout your life; and you're never too old to start.

NB During the *whisperer-loss phase*, we prefer you not to build muscle. You can and should work on that after you reach your target weight. Build muscle, get fitter and practise balance with simple tasks such as standing on one leg when you brush your teeth.

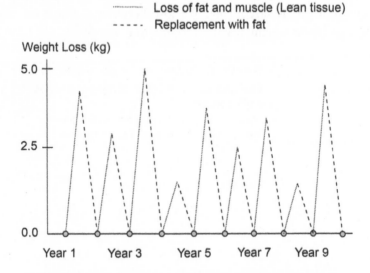

Figure 6.3. Diet failure. The Yo-Yo phenomenon. Repeated cycles of weight loss follwed by weight gain. Muscle and fat lost during the diet, is replaced by new fat as the weight returns.

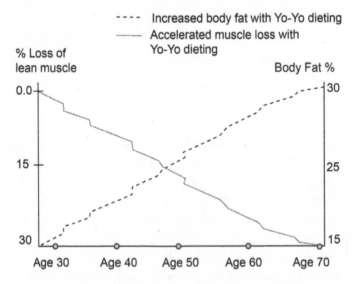

Figure 6.4. Diet failure. The Yo-Yo phenomenon. Weight loss using fad diets lose both muscle and fat. When the diet fails, fat replaces the lost muscle as well as the fat.

GETTING ENOUGH DIETARY PROTEIN

The daily recommended amount of protein is 0.8 grams per kilogram of body weight. That's 5.3 grams per stone or 0.36 grams per pound. If you want to build muscle, you will need somewhere between 1.2 and 2.0 grams per kilo of body weight: 7.95–13.25 grams per stone or 0.54–0.9 grams per pound. One chicken breast contains around 30 grams of protein. This can be used as a size guide when eating other meat and fish. It is possible to supplement protein, with whey for example, and absorb about 30 grams over an hour. Whey protein supplements come with a scoop that measures out 30 grams for this reason.

This is an important point regarding supplement proteins. There is a complex relationship between insulin and a protein messenger called MTOR (mammalian target of rapamycin). When nutrient proteins and carbohydrates are present in the blood, they both stimulate MTOR to get on with building muscle. When MTOR is higher we build more muscle. MTOR is raised most when we consume branched chain amino acids (BCAAs) and of these, the most powerful is leucine. The other two, valine and isoleucine, are also powerful simulators of MTOR and muscle repair and growth. And these supplements are available on their own, usually in the mixture 2:1:1. But as much as these may stimulate MTOR, the real lesson here is that you can only build muscle if all 21 amino acids are present.

If you eat a protein-rich meal with fats and slowly digested vegetables with lots of fibre (unrefined carbs), it is possible to absorb more than twice as much protein. Even so, if you want to build muscle then you may supplement your diet with whey protein. This has been shown to have other benefits, including reduced blood pressure, reduced abdominal circumference and reduced insulin resistance. It also reduces appetite via a series of hormones (cholecystokinin; GLP-1 and leptin, our satiety hormone) and by reducing ghrelin, our hunger hormone. So, if you don't fancy all those chicken breasts for building muscle, there is an alternative.

CHAPTER WHISPERINGS

- There are 21 amino acids, of which 9 are essential.
- This macronutrient is another string of pearls, this time with amino acids.

- Protein is found in meat, dairy and some vegetables.
- Protein and its amino acids are present in so many of the body's tissues.
- Our muscles get smaller after the age of 35; a process called sarcopenia.
- Sarcopenia is worsened significantly by yo-yo dieting, which mimics the effects that severe illnesses have on muscle mass.
- We can only absorb 30 grams in one meal taken alone; with added fibre we can absorb up to 60 grams.
- We can safely supplement with whey protein, which also reduces our appetite.
- We should build muscle as we get older.
- BCAAs will stimulate insulin and MTOR to build muscle, but this can only happen when all 21 amino acids are present.

7

GUT BUGS: YOUR FELLOW TRAVELLERS

All disease begins in the gut.
Hippocrates, 460 BC

Humans are the dominant species on the planet. We are vain enough to believe that we, at the top of the evolutionary tree, and being the cleverest species, are in control of our destiny. But the evolutionary tree is shaped more like a bush and there is no definitive top. Eagles can see eight times as far as we can, cheetahs can run almost three times faster than we can and dogs have a more acute sense of smell by a factor of 10,000. Most people would assert that we clearly win in the intelligence stakes, but how many of us could remember where we hid 3,000 nuts a season, in a woodland, like squirrels do? And do we really control our wishes and desires?

We think that we decide when we want to eat, when to stop eating and when to smile. But if I told you that this may not be quite true, would you feel slightly uncomfortable? I am not referring outwards to the reaches of alien control, but inwards to your gut bugs. They have much, and I repeat *much*, more influence over you than you may realise. Your fellow travellers, your gut bugs, have a say in what you do and how you feel. Maybe we are not as dominant as we think.

WHAT ARE OUR GUT BUGS?

You are made up of 30 trillion cells – a lot – but your gut bugs number 38 trillion cells.[1,2,3] And, while certainly outnumbered, it's hard to get a handle on 38 trillion gut bugs, but consider this:

1 million seconds is 12 days
1 billion seconds is 30 years
1 trillion seconds is 30,000 years
8 trillion seconds is 255,000 years
38 trillion seconds is 1.2 million years

So, quite a big number! And most people are unaware of their fellow travellers. Your gut bugs live in a highly interdependent community composed of microorganisms, invisible to the naked eye.

And not only are the members of the bug community highly dependent on each other, they are also highly dependent on you. Moreover, you are highly dependent on them. It is true to say that we can't live without each other.

Imagine a beautiful, diverse and colourful English cottage garden, that needs maintaining with regular watering, feeding and tender loving care. And so, your gut bug 'cottage garden' needs caring for as well. And if you look after your gut bugs, they will reward you and look after you too. Treat them badly and you will pay, with metabolic diseases, obesity and poor health. It really is as simple as that.

Humans have been living in concert with gut bugs ever since we diverged from our common ancestors over two million years ago.[4] Gut bugs found a niche market and produced things that humans couldn't, and learned to live in our guts without harming us, and we learned to feed and protect them.

The medical terms for gut bugs include gut microbiome, gut microbiota, and sometimes just microbiome, but I will use the term 'gut bugs' here, as we like this term at Whisperer HQ. Gut bugs are composed of many different species of microorganisms such as bacteria, viruses, fungi and moulds.[5] The community has certain properties, including resilience, which means that they can survive in times of adversity and one species can compensate for another, improving survival chances.

Gut bugs, being highly dependent on each other, produce food and even vitamins for other bugs.[6,7] Specialist bugs produce B vitamins, which they use themselves but also share with the community. Don't even think that we benefit from the spoils of their precious vitamin B production; bugs keep this for themselves!

The greater the number of species, the more diverse the colony and the greater the resilience.[8] Highly diverse gut bugs produce a wider range of useful substances for us than a colony with low diversity and fewer species. Dysbiosis means a sick gut bug community, characterised by loss of species and lack of diversity.

We have hundreds of different species in our gut. Some bugs are more important than others, so-called *keystone* species that keep other bugs in check. Think of it as a policing exercise; like any colony, some of the members are thugs. If keystone species are lost, the thugs run riot. Things then get a little ugly and serious health consequences inevitably follow.

One such example is Clostridium difficile colitis (C. diff), a very serious condition, with a mortality (death) rate of between 3 per cent and 30 per cent. Many people have C. diff in their guts, but it does not normally harm them, as the numbers are kept under control by the keystone species. But drugs such as *antibiotics* interfere with gut bugs. Antibiotics wipe out keystone species, allowing C. diff to get the upper hand. Then C diff rapidly multiplies, numbers grow, and toxins released by C. diff damage the lining of the colon, resulting in C. diff colitis. Faecal transplants containing healthy gut bugs can restore the balance and this is a proven successful treatment.[9] If you think that C. diff colitis is rare, think again. In the USA, C. diff colitis affects an estimated half a million people per year. It is the cause of much family trauma and grief.

Our gut bugs are found throughout the gut from mouth to anus (Figure 3.1).[10] All food is digested by your own digestive enzymes, a process finishing at the end of the small bowel. The residual matter then travels to the large bowel, where the highest concentration of gut bugs is found. There they feed on the residue – fibre! This is hopefully another Eureka moment – yes, a high-fibre diet is for your gut bugs!

Gut bugs are highly specialised, each species requiring specific growing conditions, much like the aquatic life in a river.[11,12] There are specialist bugs, who live beside the gut wall, others in the inner mucous layer and others in the middle of the gut. Each species plays a specific role in a specific place and many roles overlap, giving the colony resilience.[13]

Gut bugs respond to both external and internal stimuli; there is a lot that you can do to support them, which we will look at later in this chapter.[14]

WHAT DO THEY DO EXACTLY?

Your gut bugs produce chemicals that are useful to you, that determine your mood and appetite, and affect your health. All cells in all organisms produce chemicals via their genes. The more genes an organism has, the more chemicals it can produce, and the more powerful the manufacturing capacity.

Humans have 30,000 genes, which determine what we are made up of.[15] Genes control the supply and manufacture of chemicals that influence our metabolism.

Your gut bugs however have a staggering 22 million genes, trouncing your own meagre production capacity.[16,17,18,19,20,21] And that is why you need them; your gut bugs make chemicals you need but can't make.

Gut bugs have a major input into the immune system, mental function, mental health, gut motility, hormone production and energy metabolism.

Gut Bugs and Immunity

Immunity is central to survival and the immune system repels foreign invaders, not least Covid-19. It also needs to recognise your own tissues so that it does not attack you, which happens in autoimmune diseases. Gut bugs have a major role in both setting up the immune system in childhood, and maintaining it throughout life.[22] Inflammation is a constant finding in metabolic diseases and is linked to gut bugs, as is dysfunction of the immune system.

Gut Bugs and the Brain

'It's a gut feeling,'; of course it is, because gut bugs produce and help to control multiple hormones and neurotransmitters, such as serotonin, which affect the brain. Gut bugs have a great deal of influence on the brain, in part explaining the close, recognised association between mental disorders and gut problems.[23,24,25] And they exert their influence in two ways: either via the vagus nerve or through chemicals released directly into the blood.

Gut bugs stimulate the vagus nerve, which transmits messages directly to the brain. When I was in medical school, it was an important mantra that the vagus nerve was a one-way system and transmitted messages from the brain to the gut. Nothing the other way round; the brain was king and was the controller. Now we know this is not the case, and in fact it is a two-way neural highway that also transmits messages from your gut directly to your brain. Thus, the gut bugs influence the brain directly via the vagus nerve.

Gut bugs also make active chemicals such as GABA and other short-chain fatty acids, which are transported to the brain via the blood. One such chemical, acetate, plays a role in the central suppression of appetite by the brain; but acetate is produced by gut bugs. Now where's that free will?[26]

Serotonin is a well-known happy hormone and people with depression frequently take Prozac, which increases serotonin. More than 1 in 6 adult Americans – that's over 55 million people – reported taking psychiatric drugs over the course of one year. A truly incomprehensible number.[27] Between 10 and 20 per cent of the UK adult population take antidepressants.

But did you know that serotonin must be produced *every* day and you need daily tryptophan in your diet to produce it? And that your gut bugs help to control the production of serotonin?[28,29] Tryptophan is found in chicken, cheese, nuts, seeds and pineapple. Well, there you go; the prescription-writing doctors are hardly going to tell you to eat a diet rich in tryptophan so you can make enough serotonin. That wouldn't be good for Big Pharma's shareholders!

HOW DO THEY AFFECT MY WEIGHT?

Some years ago, pictures on the internet of a fat mouse and a thin mouse went viral. Transplanting gut bugs from fat mice to thin mice made the thin mice fat, even though their diets were unchanged. This led to widespread public interest in the role of gut bugs in weight control. People started to imagine that a faecal transplant might cure obesity but, as always, it is a little more complicated than that! It's all very well planting a beautiful cottage garden, but without the necessary TLC it soon reverts to a patch of weeds.

It has been recognised for some time that gut bug dysbiosis occurs in several conditions, including obesity and diabetes.[30,31,32,33] Recent research has shown strong links between nutrition, gut bugs and health.[34] Study subjects who ate a healthy diet had high levels of good gut bugs and a low risk of metabolic disease. Subjects who ate an unhealthy diet had high levels of bad bugs and a high risk of metabolic disease. And diet strongly affected gut bug composition.

Fifteen species have been identified as good bugs, associated with health, and fifteen more as bad, associated with insulin resistance, abnormal metabolism and obesity. These findings support the belief that altering nutrition improves gut bugs, metabolism and health and promotes weight loss.[35,36,37]

As people binge on processed food, with high amounts of sugar and HFCS, the gut bug community is eventually overwhelmed. Long-term, a Western Pattern Diet will result in destructive changes to your gut bug colony; first species loss, then loss of keystone species, then loss of diversity, and alteration in the ratio of bad to good gut bugs.

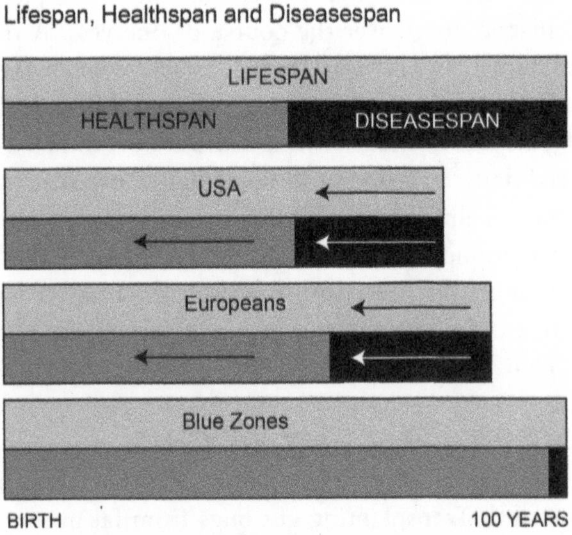

Lifespan, Healthspan and Diseasespan

Figure 7.1. Lifespan, healthspan and diseasespan in the US, Europe and the Blue Zones. The Western Pattern Diet, is lowering the age when diseasespan begins.

Eventually, the bad bugs, bloated on sugar, omega-6s and trans fats, overpower the good bugs and you will find yourself boarding the metabolic bus at the first stop: insulin resistance. Your metabolism goes awry, you gain weight and, if you keep doing what you have been doing, you will continue to get fatter and fatter. And remember, obesity is a *sign* that the metabolic 'engine' is not working properly. Unless you feed your gut bugs properly, you will stay on the metabolic bus (Figure 1.1).

HOW DO I HELP MY FELLOW TRAVELLERS?

Your diet is the single most important determinant of your gut bugs, although there are plenty of other factors (Figure 7.2). What you eat is feeding the trillions of gut bugs that live inside your gut.

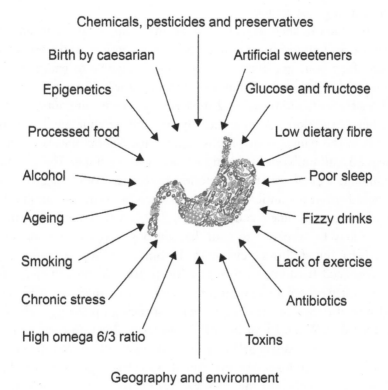

Figure 7.2. The bad influencers of gut bugs.[12,35—37]

The first way to help your gut bugs is to eliminate all the things that harm them, such as food that promotes the growth of bad bugs, including sugar, processed foods, burgers, sweets and muffins.

When you have reached your target weight, at the end of the plan, you can concentrate further on supporting your gut bugs by eating plants, lots of different plants. Experts have suggested up to 30 different plants per week is just about perfect. Adding in probiotics such as fermented vegetables, live apple cider vinegar, kefir and live yoghurts also supports your gut bug colony.

You may worry about the effect of fasting on your gut bugs, as we did at first, but, like any creature, they too like a rest and they benefit from fasting.[38] The colonies also improve with exercise; it's not just your dog that likes a run. The diversity of your gut bugs increases with your fitness; what a nice thought, off for a run and your gut bugs get fit too![39]

Other factors such as your genetic make-up, your environment, chemical and atmospheric pollutants, where you live, and your stress levels affect your gut bugs. They are quite sensitive to emotion and being in a loving relationship also improves their diversity.

Preservatives, additives, emulsifiers and sweeteners are not good for gut bugs. Antibiotics are particularly harmful to your gut bugs; the clue is in the name. 'Anti' means against and 'biotic' means a living thing. So, an antibiotic is a drug against a living thing. The gut bug community can take six to nine months to recover from a single course of broad-spectrum antibiotics. The message is clear: use antibiotics only for a serious illness and take steps to help your colony thereafter.

You may be surprised to read that gut bugs like to sleep too, and their behaviour follows a circadian rhythm.[40,41,42,43] (see Chapter 13). So, you need to sleep, so they can 'sleep' too. When you sleep the night shift workers appear, bugs that clean and munch up dead cells and bits of debris in the dead of night, sprucing up the gut tube for the next day. When I visit beautiful Singapore, I get up early to run. When I see the cleaners and cleaning machines all around the city, I think of my gut bugs. As the day dawns, the night workers like *Akkermansia* melt into the dark gut crypts and shadows, and then the big guys wake up and get going, doing their digestive thing.

Your gut bugs respond to what you do, and what you do has a big effect on them. In turn, what they do has a big effect on you. Learn to look after them; you will not regret it.

CHAPTER WHISPERINGS

- The term 'gut bugs' is our term for the gut microbiome, gut microbiota and microbiome, which all mean the same thing.
- Your gut bugs consist of microorganisms, invisible to the naked eye, and are composed of bacteria, viruses, fungi and moulds.
- Gut bugs are a highly interdependent community.
- Humans have evolved with their gut bugs over millions of years.
- Gut bugs vary in composition depending on diet, environment, geography, exercise and stress.
- Gut bugs make a variety of chemicals, necessary for your survival, that you cannot make.
- Gut bugs produce multiple chemicals such as neurotransmitters and short-chain fatty acids.
- Gut bugs play a vital role in immunity, mental function, mental health, gut function and energy metabolism.
- A healthy gut bug community has a high degree of diversity and resilience.
- There are strong links between a person's diet, their gut bugs and their health.
- Abnormal or bad gut bugs contribute to insulin resistance, metabolic syndrome and obesity.
- When you eat, you are also feeding your trillions of gut bugs.

8

GOOD FAT, BAD FAT

The lunches of fifty-seven years had caused his chest to
slip down into the mezzanine floor.
P.G. Wodehouse, *The Heart of the Goof*

It is important to think of your body fat as spiralling up or spiralling
down; it's never in a steady state. Here we are dealing not with the
fat we eat, but with our own stored body fat, the good, the bad and
the ugly. Our body fat includes:

- Subcutaneous fat: the pinch an inch variety (Figure 8.1). This helps
  to keep us warm and jiggles around when we move. It's on our
  back, our legs, in fact all over the body. Generally, women have
  more of it than men. It is an effective insulator and protective
  layer not only in us, but in marine animals such as seals and
  whales. In modest amounts this fat is not dangerous.
- Liver fat: the most active part of the fat stores. This fat is turned
  into sugar when our glycogen stores are low. It is also used to
  make ketone bodies when we are fasting.
- Visceral fat: the bad boy (see opposite).
- Intramuscular fat: the fat *within* our muscle fibres, which is a
  normal part of our fat stores.
- Marbling in your meat is caused by fat *between* muscle fibres.
  People who are obese have huge calf muscles; that's human
  marbling from eating carbs from *Big Food*. They will also be
  rattling full of pills from *Big Pharma*.
- Orbital fat: like other fats, this provides physical protection to
  our organs, in this case the eyes.
- Cell walls: every cell has fat in the form of lipoproteins in its wall.

- Neurological fat: 60 per cent of our brain and neurological tissues are fat. Yes, I said 60 per cent! Dietary fats, in the form of omega-3s, are *required* for good fetal and newborn brain development. Later in life they may also be protective against many other neurological diseases, including dementia.[1]
- Hormones: many are made from fats.
- Fat cells: also release their own hormones.
- Vitamin transport: fat-soluble vitamins A, D, E and K require fat for absorption from the gut.

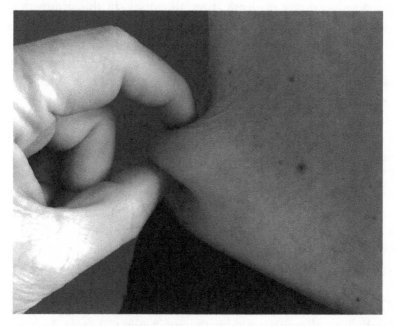

Figure 8.1. Pinching an inch of subcutaneous fat.

So, *most* fat is wonderful stuff, and intrinsic to human survival and health. The major exception is visceral fat.

BAD FAT: VISCERAL FAT

Visceral fat (VF) is the real bad boy of fat. It lies deep in your abdomen; you cannot 'pinch it', or even feel it. Quietly, surreptitiously and with great stealth it pushes out your belly from within. So, if your belt and trousers seem to be shrinking and your calf muscles are getting bigger, worry. Worry big time. Get tested and use the *whisperer reset plan* to turn things around – this is possible at any stage, at any age.

VF is present in over 80 per cent of obese people. It is also present in over 80 per cent of people in the USA who are not traditionally fat; those we call *metabolically obese*.[2] This was first recognised and named as metabolically obese normal weight (MONW) 29 years ago.[3] Big risk factors for MONW are lack of exercise, alcohol and the consumption of quickly digested carbs and high frequency meals. MONW is commonly seen in South Indians and Asians.[4]

Overweight people aged over 65, with a BMI in the range 27–29, have a reduced risk of death from all causes. In this group weight loss on BMI alone is inadvisable, but they *must* be serially investigated for abnormal metabolic markers and visceral fat and advised accordingly. We know obesity is unstable in younger people, and risks progressing to full-blown metabolic syndrome, so weight loss is recommended.[5] A recent study of 388,000 adults over 11 years showed that those with a BMI of 30 and over had increased risk of death from all causes, debunking the myth that you can be fat and healthy.[6]

Visceral fat produces so many hormones (20 identified at time of writing) that it is considered an organ in its own right. And they're bad hormones too. We are still far from knowing all of their effects on us, but I'll be willing to wager that no great news will emerge from studying this group.

METABOLIC SYNDROME

Metabolic syndrome is a combination of insulin resistance, high blood pressure, abnormal cholesterol and increased abdominal girth. The international definition is:

1. Waist >37 inches (>94 cm) in men or >31 inches (>80 cm) in women along with the presence of two or more of the following:
2. Blood glucose greater than 5.6 mmol/L (100 mg/dl) or diagnosed diabetes
3. HDL cholesterol <1.0 mmol/L (40 mg/dl) in men, <1.3 mmol/L (50 mg/ dl) in women or drug treatment for low HDL
4. Blood triglycerides >1.7 mmol/L (150 mg/dl) or drug treatment for elevated triglycerides
5. Blood pressure >130/85 mmHg or drug treatment for hypertension

CONSEQUENCES OF METABOLIC SYNDROME

Just about every non-communicable disease (NCD) can be caused or worsened by metabolic syndrome. It really is the scourge of the twenty-first century, for our health, health services and ultimately our personal and societal wealth. Without personal and government intervention it will take everything from us.

Metabolic syndrome is associated with:[7,8]

- Cancer: obesity is proven to be the biggest cause of cancer, after smoking.
- The Unholy Trinity of obesity, smoking and lack of exercise, which leads to morbidity and premature death.
- Silent death: visceral fat doesn't hurt. It causes few symptoms for many years, then health fails suddenly, leading to long-term illness and early death. It's a ticking bomb.
- Poor sleep: sleep is our biggest daily healer, relieving stresses and allowing our body to repair and regenerate. It allows the reversal of the earliest cellular changes of many types of cancer. Poor sleep is proven to be associated with shortening of our telomeres and life expectancy, worsening diabetes, ischemic heart disease, strokes, anxiety, accidents, depression, and many more (see Chapter 13).
- Snoring: causes relationship problems, as well as dry and sore throats, recurrent infections and poor sleep quality.
- Sleep apnoea: an extreme form of 'internal throat collapse' with dangerous changes in blood oxygen. Also causes afternoon tiredness and drowsiness, associated with industrial and road traffic accidents. It often requires sufferers to sleep with a mask on, puffing high-pressure air into their airways, called CPAP. Children now get sleep apnoea too; it is associated with serious oral health problems.
- Fungal infections: athlete's foot, genital candida, body crease redness, soreness and infections. Look at your own skin creases in armpit and groin; redness can be one of the first signs of insulin resistance and metabolic problems.
- Increased absenteeism from work: 7 per cent higher; from school: 54 per cent higher.[9,10]
- Psychological disorders, anxiety, depression and possibly spectrum disorders in children.

- Urinary stress incontinence.
- Gall bladder disease.
- Osteoarthritis.
- Infertility and pregnancy problems.
- Polycystic ovarian syndrome.
- Stiffness/reduced flexibility, leading to difficult toenail care and mobility.
- Regurgitation and reflux: abdominal pressure causes gastric reflux with water brash, a nasty taste in the mouth. Reflux causes changes to the lower oesophagus, with increased cancer risk. Reflux and water brash may also occur while bending to attend to shoes or feet.
- Exercise: reduced exercise tolerance, leading to a reduction in cardiovascular fitness and subsequent risks of cardiovascular disease.
- High blood pressure: hypertension is a central part of metabolic syndrome.
- Dietary salt intolerance with resultant hypertension because of sodium retention at the kidney.
- Hypertension in turn leads to cardiovascular disease and an increase in heart attacks, strokes, kidney failure and much more. Use *the whisperer reset plan* and low-grade walking exercise to *cure* it rather than pills to *control* it. And when you're better, give the book to your doctor! If every GP gave their patients the *whisperer reset plan*, it would be healthier and cheaper than the 100 million GBP we spend on uncomplicated stage one hypertension each year.
- Type 2 diabetes: leads to lethargy, cardiovascular disease, amputations of toes, feet and lower limbs, heart attacks, strokes, bacterial infections, fungal infections, reduced immunity, kidney failure, eye diseases, irreversible blindness, neurological problems, paraesthesia (numbness), peripheral neuropathy and vasculopathy leading to infections and gangrene. In men, it leads to erectile dysfunction at a much earlier age. Type 2 diabetes is occurring at younger ages and is now seen in teenagers.
- Obese babies, born to mothers with metabolic syndrome and visceral fat. Epigenetics forecasts a life of obesity.
- Reduced gut microbiome diversity and leaky gut, leading to a whole host of autoimmune diseases.

Other problems include lichen planus, SLE, psoriasis, acanthosis nigrans, inflammation, fat cell inflammation with changed CRP, IL-1, IL-6, adinopectin and leptin resistance, joint problems, rheumatoid arthritis, oxidative stress, small intestine bacterial overgrowth (SIBO), schizophrenia, tiredness, non-alcoholic fatty liver disease (NAFLD) and liver failure, thyroid dysfunction, hormonal problems, visual dysfunction, cataracts, macular degeneration, diabetic blindness, retinal artery occlusion, retinal vein occlusion, lower lid entropion; the list goes on and on.[11,12,13] Primary gout in normal weight people is also associated with metabolic syndrome.[14]

Every extra inch around your waist from visceral fat increases your cardiovascular risks by 5 per cent.[15,16,17,18]

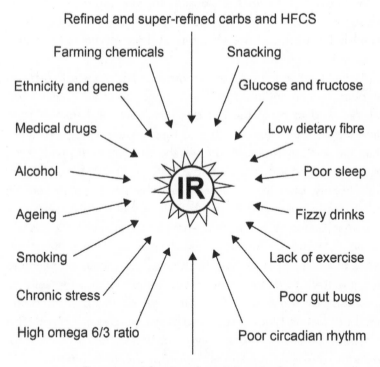

Figure 8.2. Just as the Sun is at the centre of our universe, insulin resistance (IR) is at the centre of our 'metabolic' universe.

What Causes Metabolic Syndrome?

Metabolic syndrome is such an impending disaster, societally and personally; we need to know how we got here.

Just as the Sun is at the centre of our universe, *insulin resistance* is at the centre of our personal 'metabolic universe'. In other words, we can trace back our metabolic storm and obesity to insulin resistance (Figure 8.2).

> Absence of blood insulin causes *catabolism*;
> we lose weight, as our fat cells *release* fat.
> Raised blood insulin causes *anabolism*;
> we gain weight, as our fat cells *store* fat.

We know that insulin is responsible for opening the cell 'doors' for sugar to enter fat and muscle cells for energy, or to be stored as body fat. Each cell door has lots of these keyholes for insulin to unlock.

As we trash our body with more *quickly digested* carbs, in *amount, refinement and frequency*, more and more insulin 'keys' are required to open the cell door to allow the sugar in. With time the cells become resistant to these insulin keys, and rather than the one key required to open the door normally, two, three or four keys are required (Figure 8.3). Over time it becomes ten, then twenty, then thirty. You can see what's happening here. In other words, more and more insulin is required. As a result, our pancreas becomes exhausted, and our blood insulin levels are raised all the time, even during fasting periods. Hence the importance of a fasting insulin test. Eventually, the exhausted pancreas flogging itself to death cannot meet the demand of the cells, all screaming for more keys. Then the sugar backs up in the blood and both fasting blood insulin *and* blood glucose are raised. This is type 2 diabetes. Importantly, it may take many months, or years of increasing insulin resistance for this to happen.

So, hopefully another Eureka moment for you. High-carb diets lead to insulin release, insulin resistance and fat storage. Diets high in fats don't do this! Maybe a second Eureka moment!

It is not obesity *causing* the problems; insulin resistance *leads* to obesity and then the maelstrom of other metabolic and medical problems listed above. In the initial stages, insulin resistance will exist alone, without symptoms. Later comes lethargy, brain fog and hunger (oh no). If you feel worried after looking at the diagram, insist on a test from your doctor. The blood tests to ask for are on the website.

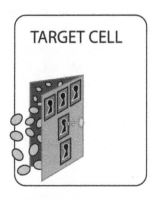
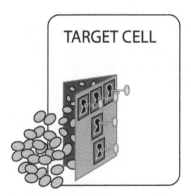

Figure 8.3. Insulin resistance. Glucose entering the cell from the bloodstream in the presence of insulin, opening the cell door. On the left is normal health, on the right much more insulin (keys to the door) is required, and the blood glucose backs up, raising blood glucose.

So: sort your insulin resistance and your metabolism and obesity will look after themselves. Be patient, take your time and everything will come right. And you get to feel great and give yourself the best chance of a healthy long life to boot!

TESTS FOR METABOLIC SYNDROME

Scans
For early detection, we need to be able to determine who has visceral fat and quantify it, then re-measure it after lifestyle changes have taken place. The gold standard test is a CT scan, but these are expensive and give you a fair wallop of radiation, making it a non-starter for repeated testing in people who want to track their progress.

The next best test is a DEXA scan, which is cheaper, correlates well with the CT scan and is 0.003 the radiation exposure, so is suitable for repeated measurements of visceral fat. Ultrasound is also effective, but must be in good hands, so is too variable.

Home testing for metabolic syndrome

There is a whole raft of anthropometric tests, measurements easily done at home with a tape measure and bathroom scales. These are 'surrogate' measures of body fat composition and include waist-to-hip ratios (WHR), waist circumference (WC) and a body shape index (ABSI).

Your body mass index (BMI) can be calculated on our website, using height and weight as the two variables. It was originally called the Quetelet index after its Belgian inventor Adolphe Quetelet in the nineteenth century as a measurement of *total* body fat. A normal value for BMI is 18.5 to 24.9, underweight is less than 18.5, over-weight is 25.0 to 29.9 and obesity is classified as a BMI over 30. Never did Quetelet imagine that we would need to reclassify the over-30 BMI into over 35, and over 40, known as morbid obesity. Because people didn't approve of the word 'morbid', BMI has been reclassified into class 1 obesity (30 to 34.9), class 2 obesity (35–39.9) and class 3 obesity (>40). In medical terms morbid means, leading to morbidity, or 'anything causing medical harm' and is not a pejorative term. Another great word lost to the thought police.

Waist Circumference (WC)

For men, a waist circumference below 37 in (94 cm) is 'low risk', 37–40 in (94–102 cm) is 'high risk' and more than 40 in (102 cm) is 'very high'. For women, below 31.5 in (80 cm) is low risk, 31.5–34.6 in (80–88 cm) is high risk and more than 34.6 in (88 cm) is very high. These are the UK guidelines for people of white European, Black African, Middle Eastern and mixed origin.

For men of African Caribbean, South Asian, Chinese and Japanese origin, a waist circumference below 35.4 in (90 cm) is low risk, and more than that is very high risk. For women from these groups, below 31.5 in (80 cm) is low risk, and anything above is very high risk.[19]

Waist-to-Hip Ratio (WHR)

Simply divide the circumference of your waist at the level of your belly button, by the circumference of your hips at the widest point. If you can feel the top of your pelvic bone on either side above your hips, that is the ideal height for a waist measurement, keeping the tape at that level all the way around your tummy. The WHO recommends for women a ratio of less than 0.85 and men 0.90. For people with a normal BMI, having a high hip-to-waist ratio doubles their risk of cardiovascular disease.[20,21]

A Body Shape Index (ABSI)

A large European study showed this to the best correlation with all-cause mortality. It showed a 30 per cent higher risk of death with high ABSI compared with low ABSI. ABSI also correlates well with total mortality, cardiovascular disease, circulating insulin, Triglycerides and LDL cholesterol.[22] As the maths and results stratifications for ABSI are a little more complex, we have an online calculator on the website, with a results guide.

DEXA

This is really our current gold standard for quantitatively measuring visceral fat. Accurate and reproducible, and will cost around 150 GBP (200 USD) per scan.

A term you may come across is the android: gynoid ratio, which is a DEXA scan ratio of fat levels between the visceral fat and subcutaneous fat. In other words, a DEXA scan version of the waist-to-hip ratio. A high ratio in children and adolescents is associated with insulin resistance and indicates a poorer health in the future for those children.[23] Worryingly, they will not achieve their full potential in school. Their life will be plagued by chronic diseases and poor health, and they will die prematurely. As a society we should be protecting our children, and we are failing them very badly.

If any of these simple tests give abnormal readings, or if you feel your lifestyle and diet are high risk, get a visceral fat DEXA scan and blood tests from your doctor. This will tell which stop you have reached on the metabolic bus, from insulin resistance to metabolic syndrome, pre-diabetes, or diabetes. No matter what age you are, and which bus stop you are at, your life is in your hands. You will come to realise that moderns medicine is crumbling under the strain of metabolic-related diseases. So, put on your blinkers and *be thine own physician*. Don't accept the *wrong tests*, or treatment of *symptoms and signs* with pills. Find the root cause of the problem and commence the *whisperer reset plan*.

MEN AND WOMEN'S FAT

Women naturally have more fat than men. Normal fat percentage of body weight is 18–25 per cent in men, increasing with age, and in women 21–35 per cent. Obesity is associated with fat >25 per cent in men and >32 per cent in women. In athletes, body fat may be as low as 10 per cent (7–13) in men and 17 per cent (14–20) in women.

FAT CELLS: SIZE, AGE AND LEPTIN

Fat cells are called adipocytes, whose number remains remarkably constant at around 15 billion throughout adulthood.[24] Turnover is remarkably low, with about 10 per cent dying and being replaced every year, and stored triglycerides on average hanging around inside the cells for about two years. When the hormone insulin is present in the blood, it causes triglycerides in the blood to enter our *existing* fat cells (see Chapter 10). In teenagers and children, the same thing happens, but additionally they lay down more *new* fat cells. So, adolescent obesity results in an increased number of fat cells for life. This is deeply shocking; our kids are being set up to fail.

And importantly, when we lose weight, fat comes out of the fat cells, making them smaller, with the number of fat cells remaining constant.

Leptin

Leptin is our satiety hormone; it tells us we're satisfied and full. It is produced by fat cells and sends a message to our brain to stop eating. The Japanese say, 'stop eating before you're full', or '*Hara Hachi Bu*'. Good strong advice from a country ranking sixth from bottom in the world rankings for obesity at just 4.3 per cent of the population.

Leptin release is greatest from fat cells that are *fewer and bigger* and lowest from fat cells that are *plentiful and smaller*, like those in an overweight teenager (another reason to prevent obesity in the young). Leptin is released 20 minutes into a meal, so slow mindful eating allows you to recognise in time when you're sated.

Note that fructose and high fructose corn syrup *directly* cause leptin resistance. You have been warned!

FAT AS AN ENERGY STORE

Our body's fuels have different energy densities; carbohydrates are 4 cal/g, proteins 4 cal/g and fat is – wait for it – 9 cal/g. So we can see that fat is our miracle store of energy. The *whisperer reset plan* will show you how to 'fat adapt' so you can burn your own fat all day long. Quite the opposite to fearing it as a food because of its calorie density. At Whisperer HQ, our mantra is

sugar makes you fat, and fat makes you thin.

BASAL METABOLIC RATE (BMR)

We all burn a certain quantity of calories daily even if we don't do any exercise. This is our basal metabolic rate (BMR). It changes with age and is different for men and women. BMR is limited as it does not differentiate between builds or levels of activity. We have a BMR calculator on the website, which you will need before starting the *whisperer reset plan*. Note: you will use the unmodified BMR, not the TEE.

CHAPTER WHISPERINGS

- Insulin resistance is the 'sun' at the centre of our metabolic universe.
- Visceral fat is known as 'belly fat' and is the dangerous fat we cannot see or feel.
- Visceral fat is metabolically active and dangerous long-term.
- Fat is an essential food.
- Differentiating between your two main types of fat is vital as a health predictor.
- The brain is 60 per cent fat.
- BMI is easily calculated but has limitations around race and build type.
- Insulin resistance and visceral fat can occur in otherwise thin individuals (MONW).
- Fat is an almost infinite store of energy, and is energy dense.
- BMR can be calculated to see our daily calorific needs.
- Other anthropometric tests are better measures of visceral fat and risk.

9

DIET MYTHS

Insanity is doing the same thing over and over and
expecting a different result.

Albert Einstein

As science has proven, both the weight loss and the other benefits
of diets are nullified after one year.[1] Diets do not work, and the
business model for most diet companies is the model of your money
being transferred to their bank accounts, quick-wins, long-term failure,
and repeat.

Let's debunk a whole pile of diet myths.

THE FIRST MYTH: DIETS WILL HELP YOU TO LOSE WEIGHT

Diets do not work. A recent meta-analysis of 29,942 patients showed
that after 12 months, benefits of short-term weight loss and metabolic
improvements had disappeared.[2] The exception was reduced LDL
cholesterol, still evident at 12 months in the Mediterranean diet (see
Chapter 5).

THE SECOND MYTH: WE BURN OFF OUR FAT

We tend to think when we burn something it disappears, but this
is incorrect. Fat has a mass and there is a law in physics called 'the
conservation of mass', which means that when we burn things they
don't disappear. The total mass of the products after 'burning' is the
same as the total mass of the reactants at the beginning. Burning doesn't
make things disappear, it merely rearranges them into other forms.

When 10 kg of fat is lost it produces some 8.40 kg of carbon dioxide (CO_2) and 1.60 kg of water.[3] Because of our hormones, and fat being converted into other macronutrients and ketone bodies, this is not quite as simple as it may seem, but the argument is largely correct. And unlike fossil fuels, you are only blowing out the CO_2 that at some point you consumed from CO_2-sucking plants, or animals that ate those plants. So, fear not; shifting a bit of lockdown lard will not cause ice caps to melt, nor polar bears to die; it's a carbon-neutral event.

THE THIRD MYTH: CALORIE COUNTING AND A CALORIE IS A CALORIE

Calorie counting, or Calorie Restricted Eating (CRE), is more accurately called the Energy Balance Model (EBM). We are told that if we reduce our calories to a level below our usual BMR, we will lose weight. This may work for a short while, but then it will fail. Think of it this way: when you don't charge your phone properly, it goes into 'battery saver mode'. With calorie restricted eating, your hormones will do the same thing to you, and you will enter 'calorie saver mode'. This is called *hormonal homeostasis*, which means 'keeping you the same'.

The argument that a *calorie is a calorie*, in the context of obesity, is simply not true, and is discussed in the next chapter.

Reasons not to do calorie counting:

1. You've started a war with your survival system, your metabolic hormones. And so, when you're in calorie deficit, they will slow down your metabolism and make you cold, tired and miserable.
2. Ghrelin increases to increase your appetite. This powerful driver will drive you mad; you'll be constantly hungry, agitated and tired. Your hormones will reduce your basal metabolic rate. You will soon adjust to your new reduced-calorie regimen, and stop losing weight.
3. These diets lower calories by mandating an unvaried and boring diet. Or even worse a diet bar filled with fructose. This can be maintained for a short while, but then the desire for other food will kick in; you will crack and go off to a burger bar. And

momentarily you will feel satiated, but then your insulin will make you feel tired *again*, and hungry *again*. The cycle of doom!

4. Calorie restricting is associated with mineral and vitamin deficiencies, reduced bone density, reduced immunity and fertility issues.

5. Fasting is a very different proposition to calorie restricting. By fasting, you are merely mimicking what our bodies have been accustomed to since humans first stood upright; times of plenty and times of fasting. And, fasting doesn't upset your hormones. In calorie restriction or small plates, or whatever fad-diet is currently fashionable, you are yelling at your hormones, 'I can beat you.' And if you shout at your hormones, they'll win. They always do, which is why the odds of any calorie-restricted diet failing are 95 per cent. Bad odds for you, but great odds for repeat business at the diet companies. Ca-ching! Fasting is not accompanied by a reduction in BMR. The ketones reduce your ghrelin, reducing any sense of hunger. The hormonal response to fasting is totally different from the response to calorie restriction. Our hormones make us perform well when we are fasting, but slow everything down when we are calorie restricting.

So, we whisper at our hormones, by mimicking scenarios they have been familiar with for generations. And guess what, they don't object and instead come happily on board. Learn to shed weight with your hormones on side, happy and contented.

THE FOURTH MYTH: THE GYM WILL MAKE YOU SLIM

Monique and I do a mix of resistance training, running, cycling and swimming. Don't get me wrong; cardio and building muscle are healthy things to do, as we discussed in Chapter 6. It's just the outrageous gym adverts that make us smile. There are four recurring howlers so spectacular, they qualify for the whisperer 'Equine Effluent Awards'. You choose your winner!

1. When people run, cycle and so on in the gym, they are taught to ADD the calories from their exercise to their normal daily BMR. Example: if your BMR is 2,000 cal per day and you do a one-hour run, burning 500 cal, you are taught your total burn

is – you guessed it: 2,500 cal. That, folks, is not how human physiology works. You see, your hormones will slow down your metabolism for the rest of the day by around 90 per cent of the exercise value. Wow, you thought two hours' running had earned you free chicken vindaloo and naan. So sorry – it doesn't work like that. The real sum has some variability, but is more like:

$$\text{TOTAL BMR (after exercise)} = [\text{DAILY BMR}] + [\text{EXERCISE CALORIES} \times 0.1]$$

In the real world of human physiology and hormonal homeostasis we get about 50 extra cal for every extra 500 (or one hour) burned through exercise. We get extra hunger, true – but we've only earned one-sixth of that naan bread!

2. We love this advert: 'what muscle building can do to boost your metabolism'. In our body the relative energy burn is: liver 25 per cent, brain 20 per cent, muscles 15 per cent; kidneys 10 per cent, heart 10 per cent; and the other 20 per cent is spread among skin, gut, lungs and fat. Muscle is about three times more metabolically active than fat. Our skeletal muscle mass is 38 per cent in men and 31 per cent in women by body weight. In a normal 70 kg man that means 27 kg in total of skeletal muscle.[4] A 10 per cent gain in this muscle from weight training would require great commitment and would result in an increase in muscle mass of 2.7 kg. If his BMR were 2,000 cal per day, his muscle burn per day would be 15 per cent, or 300 cal. This new muscle will not revolutionise his metabolism. Instead, it will burn a measly 30 cal, or one-tenth of a Snickers bar. WOW!

3. 'Afterburn from HIIT will be your saviour and burn off those calories'. Sorry folks, but afterburn accounts for very little: about 4 per cent of your BMR. Minute for minute HIIT is slightly better than cardio, but considering cardio sessions are much longer, overall effects are similar and singularly unimpressive compared to the hype. And remember, hormonal homeostasis will ensure that your metabolism goes into 'battery saver mode' for the rest of your 24-hour day.

4. There is little afterburn after resistance training. From a 40-minute session you may get 4 per cent, or 80 calories of increase over 24 hours. Wow, a quarter of that Snickers bar![5]

These are piffling amounts; our diet is by far the most powerful tool in reducing calorific balance. Please do the cardio, the HIIT and the weights, because you like it, and they're good for you. At least you won't be one of the fools believing, and even worse repeating, this bilge. During the weight loss phase of the *whisperer reset plan*, we advise continuing with whatever exercise you're already doing. If you're not exercising or doing weights, you should consider a gentle morning walk, and leave anything more strenuous until you achieve your target weight.

THE FIFTH MYTH: YOU CAN OUTRUN A BAD DIET

Let me start by saying there are some exceptional athletes who can. They are able to exercise for hour after hour and include cross-country skiers, endurance cyclists and ultra-runners. Some burn over 5,000 cal per day, which is about the maximum nutrition our gut can absorb.

I suspect by the very fact you're reading this book you're not one of them!

Unless you fall into this elite group, the more you exercise, the more your hormones slow down your resting metabolism (BMR).

So, one week you go to the gym every day and do your cardio and run for an hour on the treadmill. You're doing it well and mixing up the slow and long and HIIT, in an 80/20 plan; great for health and fitness. I know, I've done it for decades; two hours slogging my 213 pounds (97 kg) over a rotating rubber band. And in the background my hormones are sitting back, filing their nails, awaiting their moment. When I sit down in the afternoon, they slow down my resting metabolism, make me tired, fall asleep, and feel grumpy. They slow my heart rate and make me ravenously hungry. I've got one hour to beat them, and the hormones have the other twenty-three hours to make sure I lose. Yes, fat becomes more metabolically active with exercise, but just does not get burned off.[6] You have to be a very special athlete to outrun a bad diet and usually pretty lean already.

THE SIXTH MYTH: YOU CAN OUTSMART YOUR HORMONES

Your ancestors could survive harsh periods of food deprivation and were better at escaping sabre-toothed tigers than the bloke in the next cave. And on an empty belly. They could successfully hunt, and fight their enemies, also on an empty belly. If they weren't like this, they wouldn't have survived, and you wouldn't be here. So, you descend from survivors whose hormones knew how to keep them alive in times of food scarcity. You are now that person, with those same genes, and same hormones, living in a world replete with food. To reduce your body fat, you will need to become smart enough to work with your hormones, and not against them.

Hormonal homeostasis is rock-hard and stubborn as hell. Make no bones about it, in ancestral days it was survival of the *fittest*; now it's survival of the *smartest*, and you are learning exactly how to be smart.

CHAPTER WHISPERINGS

- Diets do not work if you watch them for long enough.
- Exercise doesn't work for weight loss.
- When we lose weight we breathe out our fat.
- Calorie counting does not work in losing weight because of hormonal homeostasis.
- Exercise calories are subtracted from, not added to, the daily burn (BMR).
- Afterburn from all forms of exercise is exaggerated.
- Your hormones have been keeping you safe for millennia. Work with them for total control of your weight, hitting targets and staying there.
- In ancestral days it was survival of the *fittest*. Now it's survival of the *smartest*.

10

FAT STORAGE HORMONES

Eureka, I have found it.
Archimedes

During this chapter, I promise you some Eureka moments. I'd like to start with some fantastic news. Although there are over 50 hormones, you only need to know a lot about one, and a little about another four. In this chapter you will learn why most adults can't lose fat!

In his Croonian lecture at the Royal College of Physicians in 1905, Ernest Starling, Professor of physiology at University College London, presented the word 'hormone'. Hormone is from the Greek meaning 'to set in motion', and they are quite simply chemical messengers, produced by one type of cell, that enter the bloodstream and travel to exert an effect on another distant cell. Hormones recognise their target cells by the receptors usually found within the wall of the target cell (Figure 10.1). Once they find their specific keyhole in the in the target cell, they can exert and effect on that cell. Millions of keys circulate throughout our bloodstream every day, looking for their specific target cells.

WHAT DO HORMONES DO?

Hormones modulate many of our body's functions. They regulate our development prior to birth and are responsible for ensuring we have two thumbs and eight fingers. After birth, they control our growth, start puberty, and take us through it. They control our immune system and decide who gets facial hair and who doesn't, as well as all the other sexual characteristics. The adrenal glands pump

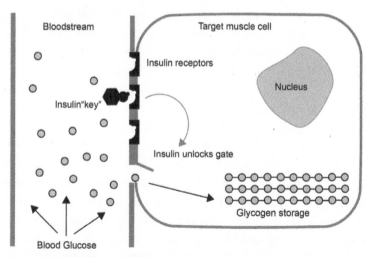

Figure 10.1. Raised blood glucose causes the pancreas to releases insulin, which binds to its receptors in the cell wall. This causes the gate to open in the cell wall, letting glucose into cells and stimulates glycogen production in liver and muscle cells. Similarly, insulin pushes fat into fat cells, increasing obesity.

out adrenaline and cortisol when we are in danger, so we can fight or flight. Our kidneys create erythropoietin, a hormone that stimulates new red blood cell production (and is on the doping list of all sports for obvious reasons). And insulin, king of hormones to any diet whisperer, is produced in the pancreas and released into the blood after we eat. It facilitates the transfer of glucose, fats and proteins from the blood into our tissues.

Our endocrine system produces our 52 unique hormones in various glands and they fly around our body at all times, doing their stuff, from controlling our blood sugar to controlling our sleep. All cells have hormone receptors, from a few to thousands. Each type of receptor is specific to one hormone type and causes the cell to perform a function. Insulin, for example (a hormone of particular interest to us), causes a muscle cell to store glucose as glycogen or fat.

INSULIN

Insulin is primarily known for its association with glucose and diabetes. But it has another vitally important function, which is fat storage. Indeed, in my medical school days it was also known as the *fat storage* hormone.

Insulin is produced in the *beta* islet cells of the pancreas. Its role is to direct macronutrients to where they are needed in the body, either to be used as fuel, or stored. When insulin finds the right receptor cell, carbohydrates, fats and proteins may enter the cell. When we consume *quickly digested* carbohydrates, they rush rapidly into the bloodstream. Insulin is released and rapidly moves sugar into target tissues. If you're exercising this may go into muscle for energy production; if you're at your desk, it will be converted into fat stores.

The sugar spike caused by quickly digested carbs is soon gone, but the insulin takes longer to disappear. Insulin was designed for slowly digested carbs, like carrots or cabbage. Therefore, as there is insulin but no excess glucose, the insulin causes the blood sugar to fall to below normal, and ghrelin is released, causing us to feel hungry again. This creates that tired, shaky, hypoglycaemic sensation 90 minutes after eating quickly digested carbs, which keeps us eating carbs, releasing insulin, and therefore constantly storing fat.

GLUCAGON

Glucagon is a close neighbour of insulin also produced in the pancreas, in its *alpha* islet cells. But its functions are very much the opposite of insulin's. Glucagon is released when blood sugar is low, to protect us from the inevitable damage that would cause. It causes glucose to be released into the blood to raise our blood glucose levels to a safe level. It does this by glycogenolysis, or the cleaving of stored glycogen into glucose units, then opens the cell gates to let it out. When liver glycogen stores run out, glucagon switches on glucose production from fats and proteins, a process called gluconeogenesis.

The actions of insulin and glucagon are *mutually exclusive*, which we look at in detail a little later.

INSULIN RESISTANCE

The metabolic bus trip is familiar to you by now. First comes insulin resistance, then obesity, then metabolic syndrome, then diabetes, then chronic ill-heath, then an early death. Brutal but true (Figure 10.2 and Figure 10.3). As insulin resistance occurs, more insulin keys are required to open the doors and let the blood glucose into the cell. Eventually, the glucose backs up in the blood and type 2 diabetes occurs.

Insulin resistance comes about with worrying simplicity and symptomless stealth. Genetics and race play a part in it, but our interaction with our food and the environment are the big external influences. So, anything that reduces the body's sensitivity to our own insulin is said to have increased insulin resistance. Increased insulin resistance is the same as reduced insulin sensitivity. They both mean the same thing.

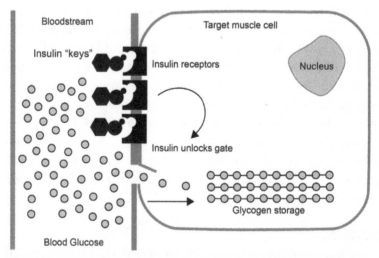

Figure 10.2. Insulin resistance. Sustained high blood glucose eventually requires more insulin to open cell gates, allowing glucose to move from the blood into cells. Blood glucose and blood insulin are levels are both raised.

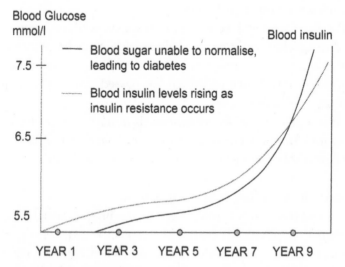

Figure 10.3. Insulin resistance over time, causing raised blood insulin, then raised blood glucose, pre-diabetes, then diabetes.

LEPTIN AND GHRELIN

Ghrelin is our hunger hormone; its release from the stomach wall triggers our brain to make us hungry. It is a powerful driver to eat more food and keep up our fat stores for leaner times. It is *decreased* by ketones, when we are fasting. It is *increased* by calorie restriction and is one of the factors that cause all calorie restricting diets to fail.

Leptin is a very important hormone, produced by gut cells and fat cells. It is our satiety hormone and tells us when we have had enough food. Raised blood sugar leads to leptin resistance as well as insulin resistance. With leptin resistance we have no sense of satiety to stop us eating. Importantly, high fructose corn syrup (HFCS45 used in food, and HFCS55 used in carbonated soft drinks), directly stimulate ghrelin and directly inhibit leptin, and build leptin resistance. Over time, this leads to many metabolic issues, cardiovascular disease and obesity.[1]

CORTISOL

Cortisol has receptors on many cells all over the body. It has an effect on our muscles, brains, lungs, heart and the rest of our endocrine system. It also affects sugar metabolism. It is a primary agent in morning awakening too (see Chapter 13). Cortisol is a steroid hormone, primarily produced in the adrenal gland that sits on its throne on top of our two kidneys.

In the fight or flight response, cortisol as well as adrenaline is secreted to quickly ready you to fight or flee. Your breath and heart rate quicken; you can sense your heart pumping. There is increased muscle blood flow. When the threat has passed, cortisol levels return to normal, over a few hours.

But it is a problem when cortisol levels *don't* return to normal but stay elevated for many hours, days or even longer-term. A chronically elevated cortisol level in our blood is bad for our health.[2]

Persistently high cortisol is associated with:
- Shortened telomeres: chronic stress is the biggest association with shortened telomeres. These are the protective caps on the end of our genes, that shorten throughout life. When they're gone you're gone too. Many aspects of the *whisperer reset plan* incorporate dietary aspects that are known to lengthen telomeres.

- Increased obesity.
- Increased visceral fat.
- Increased midline subcutaneous fat, between the shoulder blades, over the back of the neck, face and stomach.
- Insulin resistance and diabetes.
- Digestive problems.
- Muscle wasting and weakness.
- The breakdown of muscle into glucose: gluconeogenesis.
- Increased blood pressure.
- Metabolic syndrome.
- Poor sleep.
- Cardiovascular disease: heart attacks and strokes.
- Infections and immune system weakness.
- Decreased libido.
- Poor memory.
- Poor cognitive ability
- Increased anxiety.
- Reduced immune response and infections.
- Raised eye pressure.
- Glaucoma, an asymptomatic condition of raised pressure in the eye resulting in blindness if untreated.

The causes of chronically raised cortisol are:
- Medical conditions affecting the adrenal gland or pituitary gland at the base of the brain; Cushing's syndrome.
- It can be caused by steroid medications taken orally, or topically in the form of creams; yes, steroid hand creams can cause blindness in glaucoma patients.
- Oestrogen elevation in women.
- Stress and in particular how an individual responds to stress.

The ways to reduce lifestyle-related raised cortisol are:
- Learn to recognise when you are becoming stressed.
- Learn how to deal with your stress in a healthy way; this can be powerful enough to prevent heart attacks.
- Yoga and meditation.
- Spirituality (see Chapter 12).
- Be in tune with your body's circadian rhythm (see Chapter 13).
- Regular sleep patterns and sleep hygiene (see Chapter 13).

- Getting enough sleep: 6–8 hours per night for adults.
- Laughter and having fun with friends.
- Consuming enough omega-3 fatty acids.
- Good karma: try to be the best person and help others.
- Healthy diet: high in fats, medium in proteins and low in refined carbs. Plenty of fibre.
- Your partner: caressing and caring for each other.
- Stroking animals goes both ways, de-stressing you and your pet.

In Chapter 12 we will look at the most important of these in more detail.

HORMONES AND MUTUAL EXCLUSIVITY

On a cold day you put on your coat to go out. When you come in, you take your coat off. The acts of putting on and taking off are mutually exclusive. In other words, you are either putting your coat on or taking your coat off, never doing both at the same time.

Certain hormones are anabolic; that is, they cause fat to be stored and increase our body fat. Other hormones are catabolic; that is, they cause fat to be removed from the body, reducing our body fat. And these hormones are mutually exclusive; in other words, at any given time, our bodies are *either* gaining fat, or losing fat (Figure 10.4).

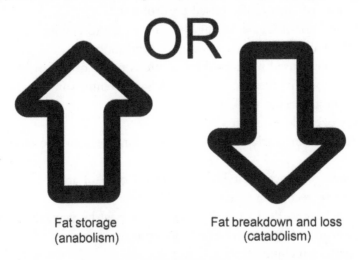

Fat storage
(anabolism)

Fat breakdown and loss
(catabolism)

Figure 10.4. Hormone driven anabolism (building and storing macronutrients) versus catabolism (breaking down or burning macronutrient stores). They are either one *or* the other and cannot co-exist. You're either storing fat or losing fat. Never both at the same time. And, if insulin is circulating, you are anabolic.

If you have circulating insulin, the major anabolic fat-storing hormone, you cannot break down fat for fuel. This point is fundamental to understanding fat metabolism. If insulin is present in the blood, you are laying down fat. So if you want to remove fat, insulin must not be present. Only when insulin is absent can the catabolic hormone glucagon start melting away your body fat.

> When insulin is around,
> fats *cannot* be broken down.
> When glucagon is around,
> fats *can* be broken down.

For a lot of people, this is when the penny drops! When insulin is circulating, fat cannot be used for fuel. After eating, insulin will be raised for two to three hours in healthy individuals and up to six hours in overweight individuals with insulin resistance, metabolic syndrome or diabetes (Figure 10.5).

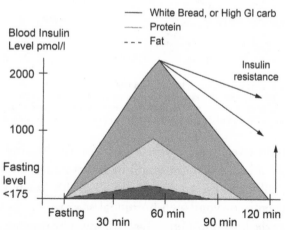

Figure 10.5. Blood insulin after carbohydrate, protein and fat. When insulin resistance, pre-diabetes or diabetes is added, the base of the insulin release widens (see arrows). It shows the differences in the amount of insulin required for different macronutrients and how much more insulin is secreted when insulin resistance is present.

All foods increase insulin. The following graph shows how different macronutrients affect blood insulin levels (Figure 10.6). And here's the rub; that chocolate digestive with your elevenses renders your body anabolic for two hours, until lunch. And then that afternoon snack before supper – the same. Before you know it, your insulin is raised 24 hours a day. Then you wonder why you're not losing any fat! It's not the number of calories. It's the *type* of food, the *timing* of the food, and the *frequency* of food. Eureka! Never let anyone tell you that *a calorie is a calorie* again.

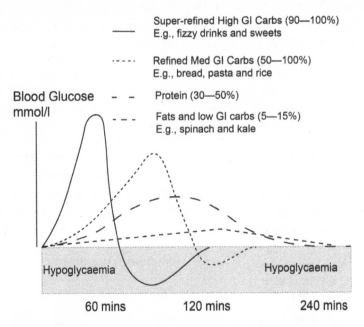

Figure 10.6. Different foods and tendancy for high and low blood glucose (hypoglycaemia) which then stimulates symptoms of hunger and re-eating. The % figure is the amount converted to glucose. Note: in healthy individuals, hypogycaemia (low blood sugar) only occurs with high GI (refined and super-refined carbs).

Your insulin levels will only be normal overnight. And even then, if you've had a bedtime snack you'll be hours into your sleep before your levels fall back to zero. I'm afraid all of this just puts you right into the epicentre of your own hormonal storm.

Fat causes the lowest insulin release, followed by protein; the highest is unsurprisingly caused by carbohydrates (Figure 10.6 above).

The corollary: what if we were to eat just one fat-filled meal a day? Say, 70 per cent fat, 25 per cent protein and 5 per cent carbohydrates. 'That much fat?', I hear you say. Well, here lies the truth: your insulin will hardly rise, and will come back to normal after a few hours.

If you want to lose weight you have to reduce your insulin. To burn fat, you must have periods when insulin is not in your bloodstream. Eat less frequently and you'll burn more fat. Eating fat causes the burning of fat. Eureka!

And with absolute certainty, cut out all forms of snacking, especially quickly digested carbohydrate foods and drinks, and 'low-fat' foods where the healthy fat is replaced by sugar.

Carbs make you fat, and fat makes you thin

PUBLIC HEALTH

You now understand the theory behind what is called the Carbohydrate Insulin Model, or CIM. In the last chapter you met the myths surrounding the Energy Based Model (EBM), otherwise known as *calorie restricted eating*, or *calorie counting*, the preferred model for the repeated failure that keeps corporate 'Big Diet' going. The EBM has been the centre of the West's public health policy. It has been an unmitigated public health failure, led by groupthink and the corporate 'Big Food' pro-sugar lobby. Government needs to press the refresh button on the stale methodology of EBM and at least look at the CIM. Whatever it takes, we desperately need it now.[3] At the Diet Whisperer, our plans also incorporate *fat adaptation* (see Chapter 11), *fasting* (see Chapter 12) and *circadian rhythm* (see Chapter 13) as these are intrinsic to long-term success in weight and metabolic control.

FIZZY DRINK SYNDROME

Too often we see obese teenagers, walking along, swinging at their side, a 2-litre (c. 4 pints) plastic bottle of a fizzy drink. They keep it close, to continuously fuel the fire of their sugar addiction, what we call fizzy drink syndrome (FDS). The teens don't know why they are trapped in this cycle of ever-increasing obesity. They don't need to eat any food to be trapped. They are not only trapped by increasing weight and fat but are also laying down new fat cells; something unique to children and adolescents. With repeated periodic drinking, insulin circulation is continuously high, locking the fat into the cells. Then hypos trigger more drinking. And the cycle goes on.

Let me terrify you with some figures. We have an orange-flavoured fizzy drink in the UK that comes in 2-litre bottles. They cost £1.85 and anyone can buy them, and sugar-addicted teens frequently do. Each bottle has the equivalent of 50 sugar cubes. Let me tell you how you can work this out simply with some very easy maths.

Fizzy drinks come with 10 grams of sugar per 100 ml. A sugar cube is 4.0 g (16 cal), and we know that 1 gram of sugar is 4 calories. So, 2 litres is 2000 ml, which is 200 grams of sugar. Multiplying by 4 gives us 800 calories in one bottle. If we divide the 200 by the weight of the sugar cube, we get 50 sugar cubes in each bottle.

A teenage girl has an energy requirement, or BMR, of 1,800 calories for the whole day. The worry about these drinks is FDS; a circular pathway: have a drink – spike your blood sugar – insulin released to chase the rise in blood sugar – blood sugar rapidly falls – insulin is still circulating, and the blood sugar falls below the normal level – and we get symptoms of low blood sugar, a 'hypo' or hypoglycemia symptoms: pallor, shakes, irritability, tiredness and lack of concentration – so we take another drink. And repeat (Figure 10.7).

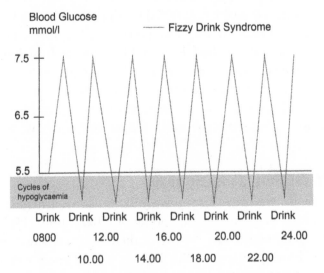

Figure 10.7. Fizzy Drink Syndrome (FDS). Recurrent spikes in blood sugar followed by recurrent hypos, stimulating the next feed cycle. Super-refined carbs in a bottle.

Even worse, the HFCS in this fizzy drink bottle directly stimulates ghrelin, our hunger hormone. The HFCS also directly inhibits our satiety hormone, leptin, and builds leptin resistance. This results in further hunger for more fizzy drinks. This is FDS and is the cycle of doom. It is refined carbohydrate addiction; it terrifies me that so many teenagers have it. Undiagnosed and untreated, it will lead to a reduced healthspan *and* lifespan. In other words, they'll constantly feel terrible, get horrible inflammatory diseases, and die early. And remember, fruit juice (see Chapter 4) does the very same thing. Fizzy drinks are more dangerous than cigarettes, and our kids can buy them with impunity. That's not liberty, it's lunacy!

CHAPTER WHISPERINGS

- Hormones are tiny chemical messengers in the bloodstream.
- Hormones attach to target cells, tissues or organs to produce a target action.
- Hormones control our metabolism.
- Hormonal homeostasis keeps us alive, but works against our efforts to lose weight
- Insulin is the hormone of fat storage.
- When insulin is present in our blood, we cannot burn fat from our fat stores.
- Refined and super-refined carbs (quickly digested carbs) lead to higher levels of insulin.
- Fizzy drinks cause hormonal havoc, metabolic syndrome, illness and premature death.
- Snacking is bad, snacking with refined carbs is worse and super-refined carbs worse still.
- Glucagon is released when healthy gaps occur between meals.
- When glucagon is increased fat is burned.
- Fibre reduces carbohydrate bioavailability and is protective against insulin spikes.
- Fizzy drinks and fruit juices are available to anyone, at any age.
- Ghrelin is the hormone that makes us hungry; its opposite number, which indicates satiety, is leptin.
- Leptin is made resistant by fructose and HFCS.
- Ghrelin was designed for times when food is scarce, not plentiful.
- Low meal frequency, and an EatSpan of under 10 hours are critical for health.
- Quickly digested carbs make us fat, and fat makes us thin.

PART TWO

THE ROAD FROM OBESITY

PART TWO

THE ROAD FROM OBESITY

The Whisperer bus, en route to weight loss and wellness

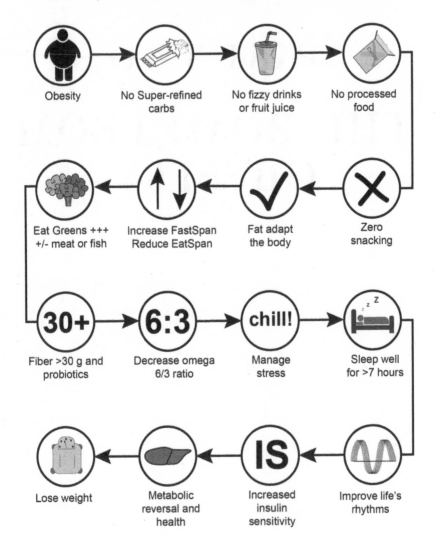

11

FAT ADAPTATION

There is only one way to survive and thrive when faced with circumstances out of our control: ADAPT.

Charles F. Glassman

Our metabolism is out of our control, addicted to carbs. As Glassman says, we must adapt. And *fat adaptation* is how we change the body from a carb burner to a fat burner. Fat adaptation is quite simply your key to lifelong wellness and weight control. To achieve this, we use two very powerful tools. Firstly, *what food*, and secondly *when food*. You will find out exactly what this means in this chapter and Chapter 12, so stick with me.

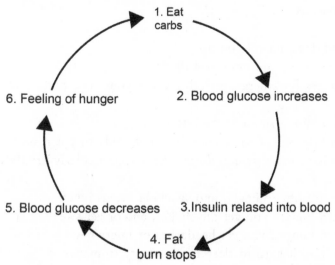

Figure 11.1. The refined and super-refined carbohydrate snacking-meal-snacking cycle of doom; turning off fat burning. The more time this happens the worse it gets, as insulin resistance builds and insulin circulates in the blood for a longer period.

During the coronavirus lockdown, I tried to buy some natural yoghurt in my local supermarket. The dairy shelves were bare except for full-fat yoghurt, all the low-fat ones having been claimed. High-fat yoghurt gives only a small rise in insulin, thereby reducing fat storage and allowing a quick return to burning fat as our fuel. (Figure 10.6). In low-fat yoghurt and other foods, the fat is replaced by carbs and the insulin release is greater, preventing us from switching on our fat burning. And we are soon hungry again.

The calorie value of fats is 9 calories per gram and sugar and protein are both 4 calories per gram. So, if you eat more fat, you get more calories: true; but look at it the other way around. We want to reduce our fat stores by using fat (which is a highly efficient source) as fuel. But first, we must learn how to *turn on* the fat-burn.

FAT FUEL INHIBITION (FFI)

This is our body's inability to switch from carbs to fat for fuel because we are addicted to the short-term rush of quickly digested carbs, a cycle repeated over and over during the day and sometimes at night (Figure 11.1). The powerful drivers of this cycle are low blood sugar and dopamine-driven addiction. See if you recognise any of these symptoms of FFI:

- Food does not fill you up.
- After meals, you often feel tired.
- You get low-energy periods during your day, particularly after lunch.
- You desire a siesta in the afternoon.
- You lose weight for a period of time, only to put it back on.
- You have mood swings during the day, particularly irritability and anxiety.
- You are often hungry, and snacking brings relief.
- When hungry you get the shakes, and/or get sweaty.
- When hungry, you get headaches or migraines.
- You find it hard to sleep on an empty stomach.
- You wake during the night feeling hungry.
- A snack makes you feel normal again.
- You get brain fog if you don't snack.

- You tend to eat carbs for snacks: pastries, cake, muffins, biscuits, chocolate bars.
- You drink fizzy drinks to satisfy your hunger symptoms.

If you recognise just one of these, you may well have fat fuel inhibition. The great news is that with a little help we can turn this around and put you back in control.

LEXUS HYBRID AND YOU

A while back, we bought a Lexus 4x4 hybrid, because I was fascinated by the idea of switching seamlessly between its two fuel sources, petrol and electricity, which it did with aplomb.

Our body can fuel itself through carbohydrates, fats or protein. Since our ancestors escaped the sabre-toothed tigers and ran miles to get food, our body knows that muscle is not only useful, but necessary for survival. Accordingly, muscle protein is spared as a fuel under most circumstances and preserved until last.

That leaves us with our two main fuels, carbs and fat. As our ancestors ran, they did so often on an empty belly. They were constantly *fat adapted*, as they hunted or evaded the tiger, as they had no quickly digested carbs to munch on. Darwin taught us, the genes from the

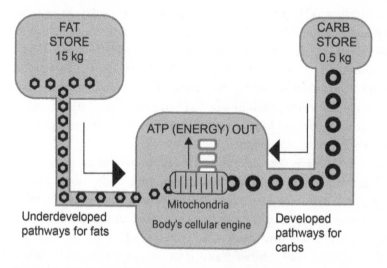

Figure 11.2. Dual fuel cellular power in the human body. Notice the narrower access from the fat stores. Fat adaptation improves the access.

losers didn't get passed on, so our metabolic systems and hormones have been inherited from the best: the winners, the survivors.

Like the Lexus, we can also switch seamlessly from one fuel to the other. The choice of fuel the Lexus uses is controlled by a microchip. The fuel we use is controlled by our hormones. So, if we live on a diet of quickly digested carbs, our insulin is raised the highest and the longest. If you eat refined carbohydrates every few hours (remember that biscuit with your coffee), your hormone insulin will be constantly raised. You are in a carbohydrate-only fuel state, unable to burn fat. Let us look in detail at the two fuel reserves that our body converts to energy (Figure 11.2).

Firstly, carbohydrate 'pearls' are re-strung and stored in the liver and muscles as glycogen. Glycogen is very rapidly available to produce our energy tokens adenosine triphosphate, or ATP. This occurs within the cell without oxygen (anaerobically) and is used by our muscles when we *begin* to move. Later, within the cell's numerous mitochondria (power stations), we use oxygen (aerobic) to burn carbs or fat. On an empty belly, glycogen stores are broken down so we continue with the carb burn. The body stores a limited amount of glycogen, around 400 g (1,600 calories). So, glycogen will last us for about 14–16 hours of fasting, or 60–120 minutes of vigorous exercise.

Secondly, fats. In contrast to carbs, fat stores around 135,000 calories in our body (Figure 11.3). As triglycerides are oxidised, they also produce ATP. This *is* fat burning. This fat oxidation is a slower process, and roughly speaking we get 20 per cent more energy from carbs than we do from fats per litre of oxygen inhaled. Give our hormones a free choice and they'll take the carbs, the fast and easy option. And when we set up this cycle of eat carbs, snack carbs, feel hungry, snack carbs, carb lunch, feel hungry, snack carbs, there is no good reason for our hormones to change, and over time our ability to burn fat decreases (Figure 11.1).

Our bodies are very adaptive. This is good and bad; think about walking or jogging. If you train correctly, your body soon adapts, and the exercise becomes easier. The downside is that in going from being *fat adapted* to *carb adapted*, our body enzymes necessary for fat burning have become fewer and weaker. So, when we first try to burn fat, we find we are fat fuel inhibited and it makes us feel terrible. We must build up these enzymes, so we are just as comfortable on either fuel.

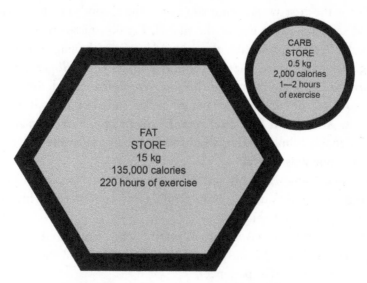

Figure 11.3. Relative amounts of fat stored and carbohydrate stored in the human body. The carb stores allow for just 1—2 hours exercise before refuelling is required, whereas the fat stores allow us to excercise for many days.

FAT ADAPTING OUR BODY

Fat adaption is the first secret to ridding ourselves of excess fat. For the past 100 years we have consumed too much super-refined and refined carbs, at too high a frequency, downgrading our ability to burn fat for fuel.

Whenever we run our carbohydrate stores down, we start to feel trembly and weak. We get some or all of the symptoms of FFI outlined above. The very moment we are about to switch our engine from carb-burning to fat-burning, we prevent it by having a cup of tea, or a biscuit. Or a slice of toast, or cake. This is how we entered and how we stay in the fat trap, where we neither eat it nor burn it.

None of this is helped by Big Food corporates and by governments who don't intervene. And you have every right to be angry about this. But channel that anger. Use it to do the opposite of what their adverts tell you. You can beat them, and we'll show you how.

FAT ADAPTATION IN TWO PHASES

There is nothing really complicated about fat adaptation when you understand the basics. What you mustn't do is confuse *uncomplicated* with *easy*. I can tell you honestly, I found it pretty rough! Really rough for the first week, quite rough for the second; but by week 4 I could see light at the end of the tunnel. I really started to feel great by weeks 7 and 8, and had the added benefit of having lost nearly 10 kg. Ask your loved ones to support you, as you *will* get irritable and irrational. Some people get flu-like symptoms (called 'keto flu'), some stomach upsets; others have brain fog and sleepiness. It will be worth it. And if you fail, dust yourself down and start over. As the famous coach John Wooden would say, 'When you wake up, make this day your masterpiece.'[1]

The time frame is highly individual, but the first phase will take between two and four weeks depending on your current lifestyle, fitness and dietary habits.

And while good levels of fat adaptation can be achieved in weeks or months, the last 10–20 per cent may take over 12 months (we know from personal experience).

There are two distinct phases to fat adaptation: *phase 1*, the high-fat diet, and *phase 2*, high-fat plus increasing FastSpan and Reducing EatSpan. If you are a bacon and egg sort of person, or a steak eater, we suggest you stay on those fats. If you're on a Mediterranean diet high in MUFAs and PUFAs, stick with those, or like us, eat a combination of both.

Fat Adaptation Phase 1:

This is the *what food* part, where we adopt a ketogenic diet to springboard into fat adaptation. The details come later, so just enjoy reading this for now.

- Start by adopting a ketogenic diet, with a maximum of 25–50 grams of carbs each day.
- Carbohydrates will be 5 per cent; fat will be 70 per cent, and proteins 25 per cent.
- You can calculate macronutrients in grams on the website.
- Eat three meals per day and never snack in between.
- Be prepared for the symptoms of 'keto flu' as your body initially struggles without the refined carbohydrate 'hits'; you are effectively going cold turkey on refined carbs.
- Stick with it; only when you have detoxed from your carbs

---

will your hormones be back in regular working order. In an emergency eat an apple, but better still try to ride the storm.
- Talk to your family and tell them what you are doing because at times you will be irritable and difficult.
- Don't weaken and have that carb hit. You need real strength in the first few weeks.
- Continue with phase 1 until you have 4 weeks under your shrinking belt.

Fat Adaptation Phase 2:

This is the *when food* part, when you learn the benefits of time-restricted eating.

- On your second four weeks the *what food* is the same, but here we start to increase the FastSpan and reduce the EatSpan, laid out for you in the whisperer plans later.
- So, on days off work, we suggest you take breakfast later.
- Try combining breakfast with lunch as a brunch.
- If you feel after a while that you can skip breakfast, then do, and have a two-meal day.
- Stick to trying to eat brunch later and your evening meal earlier.
- Eating your evening meal just one hour earlier increases your overnight FastSpan significantly.
- Every little bit of progress helps with your fat adaptation.
- Why not just eat your bacon, eggs and mushrooms for lunch? You're a real winner 😄.

At this stage you will be well on your way to being *fat adapted*. Your hormones and enzymes are now recovering and getting back to their normal state. You will be guided through all this in due course; for now, continue reading.

FAT ADAPTATION AT THE CELLULAR LEVEL

When we fat adapt, over time our cells undergo changes. Mitochondria are our cellular power stations, tiny organelles lying in the body of our cells, or cytoplasm, producing our ATP energy tokens from oxidative (aerobic) metabolism. They do so with either fats or carbs and are central to our health and wellbeing.

Like all organelles, our mitochondria naturally become old and are continually replaced. This process in cells is known as autophagy or, specifically for mitochondria, mitophagy. This replacement cycle depends on your age, genes, fitness and whether you exercise. For some people, their mitochondria will become fat adapted in 2–4 weeks, while in others it may take several months. Fat adaptation increases the size, turnover, efficiency and number of mitochondria. When you are fully fat adapted, mitochondria in all your cells will be happy burning fats as well as carbs. Your hormones will be better balanced, and you will be feeling on top of the world. Your insulin will be raised less, and raised less frequently. Your brain will also be adapted to life on 70 per cent ketone bodies. Your body and brain are now fully adapted to your new low-carb diet, fasting and cessation of snacking.

There is no magical test to tell you when you have started to fat adapt or when it is completed, but you will see the following useful signs that you are fat adapted:

- Your brain will be clear, cognition and memory improved.
- Hunger will have disappeared or be very much reduced.
- After a meal you will feel full and satiated.
- You will no longer suffer carbohydrate and junk food cravings.
- You will lose that tired feeling after lunch.
- You will have increased exercise endurance.
- You will have increased energy levels.
- You blood pressure will be lower.
- Your resting heart rate will be lower.
- You will sleep better, deeper and longer.
- You will weigh less.

CHAPTER WHISPERINGS

- The degree to which food turns off fat burning is dependent on its effect on insulin.
- Low-fat foods that are carbohydrate-enriched elevate insulin.
- Humans have a dual fuel system; we can fuel using either fats or carbohydrates.

- Muscle protein is last to be used for fuelling because of its importance.
- Carbohydrate diets with refined and super-refined carbohydrates switch off fat burning as a fuel.
- Eating carbohydrates is what makes us fat.
- Eating fats allows subsequent fat burning and allows us to lose fat.
- Diets of refined and super-refined carbohydrates are killing us and making us ill. We have become carbohydrate lemmings heading for the cliff of metabolic misery.
- Fat fuel inhibition reflects the inability to use the fat fuelling system.
- Fat fuel inhibition reflects our body's addiction to carbohydrates.
- Fat fuel inhibition can be reversed in 2–4 weeks.
- Fat adaptation is the secret to losing fat.
- Fat adaptation has two phases.
- Fat adaptation, while simple to follow, can be tough; get family or friends to support you.
- The time required for fat adaptation depends on your diet, fitness and lifestyle.
- In the early stages of fat adaptation, you may have irritability, mood swings, brain fog and flu-like symptoms. These will disappear completely once you are fully fat adapted.

12

THE ANCIENT PRACTICE
OF FASTING

To starve is to die, to fast is to live.

Herbert J. Shelton, 1950

The ancient practice of fasting is a sensible addition to the Diet Whisperer plan as it ramps up your fat adaptation (see Chapter 11). And, fat adaptation makes fasting possible, easier and more enjoyable. So, fat adaptation and fasting are symbiotic; they help each other, and over time each grows stronger and stronger. In this chapter we will also learn exactly what happens to our body over a timeline of fasting.

We saw in Chapter 9 that fasting is completely different from calorie restriction. Intermittent or periodic fasting involves periods of 12 hours or more when no food or drink (except for water, of course) is taken. Fasting periods are interspersed with meals that are not calorie 'reduced'. That said, use the website calculator as a guide to your macronutrient allowances in grams, which will reduce weekly as your weight falls.

THE BENEFICIAL EFFECTS OF FASTING

In calorie restriction, hormonal homeostasis slows the body down, as described in Chapter 9. In fasting, your hormones react in a totally different way. Instead of shutting your body down, they allow *repair* and *regeneration*. Fasting increases your stress resistance, suppresses inflammation, and improves blood glucose regulation. It also improves immunity, and all these health benefits carry over into the fed state.

This has the effect of improving mental and physical performance and increasing resistance to disease.

Specific benefits include, but are not limited to:

- Reduced weight.
- Reduced visceral fat.
- Reduced insulin levels and insulin resistance.[1]
- Reduction in all the features associated with metabolic syndrome including bad cholesterol.
- Increased Human Growth Hormone (or somatotropin), increasing fat burn directly on fat cells.[2]
- Increased autophagy, mitophagy and brain cell reparation.
- Increased cognition, short-term memory and clarity of thought.
- Reduced inflammation in many long-term conditions, such as asthma.[3]
- Reduced gut inflammation and increased gut motility.
- Reduction in blood pressure and resting heart rate.
- Activation of sirtuins, in a similar way to resveratrol, reducing oxidative stress and increasing mitophagy.
- Increased gut microbiome diversity.

There are many misconceptions about fasting. You will come across many of the common ones, so I have prepared a few lines to dispel people's worries.

COMMON MISCONCEPTIONS ABOUT FASTING

In the 21st century, we have lost many of the vital links with religious fasting, and our forefathers' healthy fasting habits. The result is a generation who think that fasting is unnecessary, uncomfortable, even dangerous. Thus, during a fast, I keep schtum, so avoiding a tirade of pseudoscience, prejudice and ignorance. You might do the same too!

1. Multiple small meals spread out across the day turns up metabolism and is best for weight loss. **Wrong**. It inhibits fat burn. It is by reducing EatSpan and lengthening FastSpan that we increase fat burn and weight loss.
2. Missing a meal puts the body into starvation mode. **Wrong**. It is

calorie restriction that puts our hormones into starvation mode, making us cold, hungry, sleepy and miserable, and turning down our metabolism. Fasting causes none of these symptoms.

3. Breakfast is the most important meal and gets your metabolism going. **Wrong.** Breakfast breaks the benefits of the overnight fast. (More on this in Chapter 21).

4. Fasting causes hunger. **Wrong.** Fasting actively prevents hunger. Hunger gets worse with calorie restriction, multiple small meals, and eating quickly digested carbohydrates.

5. Fasting causes harm. **Wrong.** Our bodies were designed to fast, and we survived intermittent fasting for 200,000 years. Fasting improves general health indicators, slowing and reversing ageing and disease processes. It promotes mental and physical health. It is highly correlated with human wellness and longevity.

6. Fasting causes cell damage. **Wrong.** Fasting is associated with healthy cell renewal, reduced ageing, and the positive effects of mitophagy and autophagy.

7. Fasting can harm our brain as our brain needs dietary carbohydrates. **Wrong.** Our brain can survive happily on the glucose and ketone bodies manufactured by the liver for us during fasting. Fasting in fact gives the brain an opportunity to detox. Current research is looking at the benefits of fasting for epilepsy and dementia.

8. Fasting will upset blood glucose. **Wrong.** Insulin levels and insulin resistance are reduced and fat burning increased, with major improvements in blood glucose regulation.

RELIGION AND FASTING

In all major faiths, fasting has played its part for aeons. For Jews, a 25-hour fast for Yom Kippur. In Christianity, Jesus fasted for 40 days and 40 nights, as part of his spiritual preparation, which is now observed during Lent. Roman Catholics refrain from meat on Fridays and remember the life of Jesus and the Virgin Mary. They also practise sobriety, contemplation and abstinence. In Buddhism, monks fast from lunchtime through to breakfast, while followers practise mindful eating: touch each pistachio nut, look at it in your hand, smell it, imagine where and how it was grown, then eat each one slowly, realising its true pleasure. The antithesis is eating in front of the television, when we may reasonably ask, how many pistachios do we remember eating? Ramadan, the ninth month of the Islamic calendar, is when Muslims fast from dawn till dusk. The meal that follows is a joyous time for family, friends and togetherness. In Hinduism, coinciding with phases of the moon, Ekadashi is practised twice monthly and worship of the god Ganesh, spiritual contemplation and fasting are observed. Arguably the most famous Hindu, Mahatma Gandhi, said, 'where there is distress that cannot be moved, my religion teaches me to fast and pray.' With knowledge, we can master our strong hormonal drives. And once again, we can take control of our destiny.

KETONE BODIES AS OUR FASTING FUEL

The ketone bodies beta-hydroxybutyrate (BHB) and acetoacetate (AA) are produced by the liver from fats, when our glucose is in short supply, at the behest of the hormone glucagon (see Chapter 10). Not only can our brain *survive* on these (90–95 per cent of the brain can utilise ketone bodies), it can positively *thrive* on them. When metabolised for energy in our brain, they produce less oxidative stress than when it uses glucose alone. So, when we switch to ketone bodies, we are helping to detox our brain! There is much promising research emerging on the role of ketones in the treatment of Parkinson's disease, epilepsy, dementia and other neurological conditions.

We have established that we do need some carbohydrate, specifically glucose, for part of our brains and all of our red blood cells. And we need this to be available 24/7. But we do not need this glucose to come from food. Our hormonal homeostasis saves us yet again. When we fast or do not consume dietary carbs, the hormone glucagon kicks into action and we start to live off the fat of the land; or more accurately off our copious fat stores in the liver and throughout the body (Figure 11.3). Our hormones keep our blood glucose within the normal range 24/7. Instead of dietary glucose, we chop off a glucose unit from our liver glycogen and send it into the blood, a process called *glycogenolysis* ('cutting the glycogen bonds'). This lasts for 8–15 hours, until the 100 grams of stored liver glycogen is depleted.

To prevent a fall in blood glucose at this point is where things get interesting; a process of glucose production from non-carbohydrates commences. This process is called *gluconeogenesis* ('glucose-new-creation') and it maintains our blood glucose by producing glucose from fats and proteins. Once again, we see that our brain and red blood cells can be maintained safely, by the upregulation of gluconeogenic hormones, which upregulate the enzymes when needed. And no carbohydrates are required, dietary or stored.

In a fasted state gluconeogenesis will happen on day 2. On day 3, our liver will begin to produce the ketone bodies. Our breath becomes 'sickly sweet' with the smell of ketones, and we have reached a ketogenic state.

During intermittent fasting:

- We must maintain our blood glucose within strict levels every minute of every hour of every day, and we can do this without dietary carbohydrates.
- Our brain and red blood cells initially use glucose from stored liver glycogen.
- Our brain and red blood cells can later use glucose produced by gluconeogenesis, using fat and protein.
- Eventually we reduce our brain's energy requirement for glucose by 90 per cent, as it switches to ketone bodies made in the liver from fats.

TERMINOLOGY OF FASTING METABOLISM

Glycolysis: glucose to pyruvate (usage of glucose for energy production)

Gluconeogenesis: pyruvate to glucose (glucose is made from other macronutrients)

Glycogenesis: glucose to glycogen (glucose units linked together for storage as glycogen)

Glycogenolysis: glycogen to glucose (breakdown of glycogen to simple units of glucose)

The first thing to say, as always, is discuss this with your doctor, who will be able to support your plan to get lighter, fitter and healthier. Talking to your doctor is also a must if you are on any medications or have any co-existing diseases. For example, diabetes or hypertension may require a reduction or even a cessation in treatment, and it must be your doctor who guides you through this reduction in treatments. How exciting would that be!

HOUR BY HOUR, DAY BY DAY: HOW OUR BODY REACTS TO FASTING

First Four Hours
The macronutrients fat, carbs and protein are broken down by digestion into their constituent parts – fatty acids, sugars and amino acids – and then absorbed from the small gut into the bloodstream. As we have seen, all three macronutrients can be stored as fat. Insulin will mediate this. Insulin also mediates the building of muscle, with any spare amino acids being stored as fat. So, our normal fed state is one of circulating insulin, with glycogen stores fully replenished. Our insulin peaks and then fades back down (Figure 10.5 and Figure 10.6).

Our glucose is now stored away, and the circulating blood glucose falls into the normal range. Without more food the circulating, blood glucose gets slowly used up. But, should this go on, the blood glucose would fall to dangerously low levels. To prevent this, the pancreas releases glucagon, increasing the blood glucose.

4–11 hours
Here we go from the storage of glucose (insulin-mediated) to glycogen breakdown (glucagon-mediated). This maintains our blood glucose in spite of the glucose 'pull' from our red blood cells and brain. At only 2 per cent of our body mass, our brain uses 20 per cent of the body's daily energy burn. That is 400 calories, equating to our whole glycogen liver stores of 100 grams.

NOTE: the 300 grams of glycogen stored in skeletal muscle is not available for this purpose but continues to be available for locomotion.

This happens on our 'natural' fast from supper to breakfast. So, glucagon keeps our blood sugar ticking along from our glycogen stores. It also is able to top up this process by gluconeogenesis. Most cells can use fats and proteins for energy directly; the brain and red blood cells are exceptions. Thanks to glucagon, blood glucose is always available for them.

If we eat now, the cycle starts all over again. If we continue to fast, then:

After 12–48 hours

The glycogen stores are depleted, and our hormones now switch us into full ketogenesis, meaning 'ketone-making'. The ketone bodies produced are acetone, acetoacetate and beta-hydroxybutyrate. The brain now switches to 70 per cent ketone use for its energy, using 280 calories from ketone bodies AA and BHB, which can, unlike other macronutrients, cross the blood–brain barrier. Simultaneously, gluconeogenesis continues producing new glucose from fats and amino acids as required. This can trickle out 80–100 grams of glucose per day into our blood, equating to 320–400 calories. Our body maintains a beautiful balance through hormonal homeostasis. It's how we've lived for 200,000 years and our genes have encoded us with the ability to fast and thrive. Fasting is a time for *repair and regeneration*, followed by feasting, where we have *building and growth*.

After 2–5 days of fasting

Circulating insulin deceases significantly, by 20–30 per cent, and ghrelin (our hunger hormone) decreases day on day, resulting in much less hunger. Repeated fasting will not only reduce insulin resistance, but also our chance of developing metabolic syndrome and type 2 diabetes. At the same time, there is a reduction in insulin resistance and leptin resistance. Autophagy will increase, replenishing our cells and making our gut and skin healthier. Our immune system cells are renewed. Autophagy is associated with slowed ageing. This may, particularly in men, produce skin shrinkage as the weight comes off.[4]

YOUR WHISPERING REGIMEN

Diet whispering is not only about whispering to your hormones, but also self-empowerment, putting you back in charge. It's about sustainable, as well as quick, results. It allows you to develop the skills you need to keep your hormones working with you, helping you achieve your metabolic and weight goals. No longer will your hormones be in charge of your fat stores. You will be in control of your hormones, and hence your fat stores, allowing you to target your weight, get there and stay there.

Once you have completed the *12-week whisperer reset plan*, you will be able to form your own regimen, based around the *whisperer-stable plan*. Alternate-day fasts, one or two meals per day, or three- or four-day fasts once a month. There is no right way, no wrong way. You can see what suits you. I know that during my three-day fasts I feel great on day 2 and better on day 3. Not hungry at all, clear of mind and feeling on top of the world. There will be a combination that suits you, and that you will come to love. And your new waistline will please you too!

SUPPLEMENTS

When Monique and I fast, we do not drink anything but water, black tea or coffee, and ensure that we take 3 litres minimum of fluids every 24 hours. I tend to monitor my intake by thirst and ensuring my urine is no darker than a light straw colour. Darker means possible dehydration. If this happens, drink more. We do not use supplements during fasting itself, as they can increase insulin and break the fast. However, we do use multivitamins, cod liver oil, calcium and vitamin D at the end of each fasting period and on non-fasting days.

CHAPTER WHISPERINGS

- Fasting is an ancient practice that we have lost connection with.
- Fasting is a part of all major religions.
- Fasting is a great way of connecting with your spirituality.
- Fasting is deeply rooted in, and related to philosophy.
- Fasting is not dangerous.
- Fasting is associated with positive changes in our brains.
- Fasting improves cellular health and turnover, mitophagy and autophagy.
- Fasting benefits the gut microbiome.

- All three macronutrients can be used to produce glucose to protect our red blood cells and brain.
- 80–90 per cent of our brain can survive on ketone bodies with just 10–20 per cent requiring glucose.
- With three litres per day of fluids we can fast safely for days or even weeks.
- Fasting should only be attempted after you have fat adapted (see Chapter 11).
- Supplements as outlined above are helpful.

13

THE RHYTHM OF LIFE

When sleep puts an end to delirium, it's a good symptom.

Hippocrates, 400 BC

All life on Earth is tied to the sun and the Earth's rotation and life takes its cues from this rhythm. We call this *circadian rhythm*, from the Latin 'circa' meaning *around*, and 'diem', *the day*. Circadian rhythm is the time control for all our biological processes. Our behaviour, and the underlying chemical reactions needed to make these behaviours happen, are coordinated. Circadian rhythm synchronises both our internal and external behaviour to the Earth's daily rotation.

Life evolved to maximise survival chances within the rhythm of Planet Earth. Some creatures adapted to the night, some to the day, and as their evolution continued, specialists within each time frame separated from other specialists. Competition, followed by differentiation made us live and function during different parts of the 24-hour daily cycle. Animals, plants, bugs and humans all have circadian rhythm.[1] Even slime mould, a brainless form of life that slithers and pulses on the forest floor, has circadian rhythm.

We are blessed with long summer evenings, and what greater pleasure than to share a glass of wine with friends and family? And where better than the garden, with the sun setting, as roses and jasmine release their intoxicating fragrances? Such plants have genes which are turned on at night, producing fragrant oils, which waft on the breeze, attracting their nocturnal pollinators. All plants need pollinators, and some have evolved to attract the night-time workers, toiling after the heat of the day. The night phlox, flowering all night with an intense aroma, is a specialist in the attraction of its pollinator, the night-flying hawk moth.

In response to *circadian rhythm*, and controlled by their plant clocks, we discover that plants can tell the time too!

Some animals live during the day and others at night. You can't change an animal's behaviour in this regard. Their clocks have evolved to sync with the day or night, as their genes, chemical processes and behaviour are tied to that part of the day. Most owls are nocturnal and if you awaken an owl during the day, it won't hunt, and it won't eat. In the day, it wants to sleep; that's the way its body clock works. You can't change its body clock. That's why it's cruel to have owls at shows during the day; like a grumpy teenager in the morning, their body clocks are set for another time.

Gut bugs (see Chapter 7) have circadian rhythm; over the course of 24 hours the composition of the colony changes, as does their function and activity. So, our gut bugs have clocks and can tell the time too.[2] *Akkermansia*, a great bug associated with health, cleans the gut lining at night, but is nowhere to be seen in daylight hours. *Crosstalk* means that gut bug rhythm influences us, and in turn, our circadian rhythm influences them.

When our ancestors discovered fire, it gave us light, and we lengthened our day. Electricity had an even bigger effect and now 'day' light can go on for 24 hours. We stretch our body clocks to the absolute limits; jet lag, shift work, erratic sleep patterns, and late-night eating, all pushing our control systems to breaking point. But there is one place that is a bridge too far, Mars. Elon Musk would have us live, work and commute to Mars. And we may well need Mars if we continue to abuse our beautiful planet. But there is one big stumbling block, our circadian rhythm. Our Earth-day is approximately 24 hours, but the Martian day is some 40 minutes longer. Doesn't sound like a big deal, but we can't adapt our body clocks to the Martian day. And that folks, is why we can't be Martians. On Mars, our metabolism would collapse, and we would slowly die. So, Mr Musk, you will need to persuade the genetic scientists to lengthen our body clocks. Good luck: 4 billion years of evolution will be difficult to unpick.

YOU'VE GOT RHYTHM

Every single one of the 30 trillion cells in your body has a clock.[3] Yes, all those body clocks are ticking away as you are reading this.

Your local cellular clocks call time in the immediate vicinity, both day and night. Each cellular clock ticks in harmony with the others, controlling your biology, from the times you sleep, to the times you eat. Your clocks are critical to life itself. Your genes have their own internal clocks, and every gene has a circadian cycle, with thousands of genes turning on and off at different times, in a cyclical fashion.

Your body clocks have an innate timing, born to tick with Swiss precision. No prompting from your brain or the outside world is required. Researchers have spent months alone in bunkers, or caves in France and Texas.[4] They discovered that the innate timing of our body clocks is approximately 24 hours; even isolated from all light and external cues, their sleep–wake cycle kept the same timing.[5]

Your body clock instinctively measures your day, reflecting the 24-hour rotation of the Earth. The healthy folk in Ikaria in Greece (one of the world's Blue Zones, discussed a little later) don't wear watches. They live with the natural rhythm of life, the sun, the moon, the stars and their body clocks.

Types of body clocks

There is a *master clock* located within your primitive brain, in a structure called the suprachiasmatic nucleus. The master clock synchronises all your *organ clocks* and *cellular clocks*. It is the central player in circadian rhythm.

But every organ has its *own* clock, with its own innate rhythm, and they can walk to the beat of their own drum. Within each organ, the level of sophistication is spectacular; thousands of genes turn on and off at different times in a synchronised fashion. And this rhythm affects not just a few genes, but 20 per cent of them.[6]

Influencers (zeitgebers)

External influencers of our body clocks (zeitgebers, pronounced zite-gay-ber) adjust the 'on' and 'off' buttons and the timing of clocks. Different body clocks respond to different external influencers, a bit like the difference between Instagrammers and Facebookers! The main influencers are *light, food, food timing* and *exercise*. Plants have relatively simple zeitgebers, influenced by light and temperature. Our bodies are a little more complicated, and internal influencers are *confounded* and sometimes *conflicted* by external influencers, such as our daily activities (Figure 13.1).

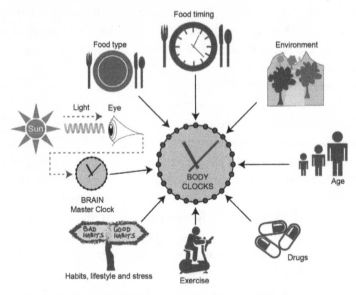

Figure 13.1. The external influencers or zeitgebers of our body clocks.

The chief zeitgeber: light

Light is the most powerful external influencer, and with over 7 billion followers, it's a big one! Light tells your master clock when it is day, and when it is night. If the master clock receives a message that there is light, this is interpreted as day, and your body gets the *wake-up* signal. If there are no light messages, the master clock signals night, and your body gets the *go to sleep* signal. The *master clock* relays messages about the light–dark cycle to *all your body clocks*, each and every day.

Only in the last 20 years have we discovered how light is processed in the eye. Hitherto, we believed that rods and cones detected light, relaying a message of day or night to the master clock; but we now know this is not the case. New findings were to prove a breakthrough and to help millions of people with their *sleep*.[7,8,9] A additional *retinal light sensor* composed of melanopsin was discovered. This sensor responds only to *blue light* and gives the master clock the *light or dark* message.[10,11,12,13,14]

When melanopsin is activated by blue light, a signal is sent to the brain saying that light is present, and the brain calls this daytime, irrespective of whether it is actually day or night. There is no differentiation between blue light from the sky, and blue light from your television, computer or phone screen.

Some years ago, sleep scientists discovered that light from our screens was having a deleterious effect on sleep.[15] Due to this work, night mode is a default on the screens of electronic devices. Millions of people have benefited directly following the discovery of melanopsin and the effect on the master clock. Night mode is a dim light, with reduced blue light, which allows your master clock to call night, helps your body clock synchrony and allows you to sleep better.

WHO SETS THE TIME?

Time is central to our lives; we (rightly) place enormous value on measuring time for all aspects of life, and the timing of our biological processes is no different.

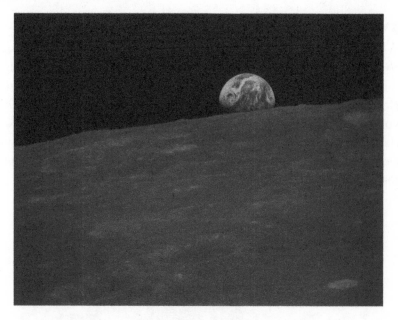

Figure 13.2. Earthrise. Apollo 8, December 24th, 1968. William Anders; 'Oh my God, look at that picture over there! There's the earth coming up. Wow, that's pretty.' Photograph courtesy of NASA.

The great captains of exploration became lost at sea with disastrous consequences, because they could not accurately measure time, and hence longitude. As more ships sailed, the wealth of nations floated, and in many cases sank, on the oceans. Longitude was of such importance, that an act of parliament, The Longitude Act, was passed in 1714. H4, Harrison's revolutionary clock, by measuring time accurately, allowed true measurement of longitude, for which he won the longitude prize. H4, his original clock, can still be seen in the Royal Observatory in Greenwich, London. Later that century, my own seafaring forefathers were able to successfully navigate the Atlantic Ocean. They would have marvelled at my wristwatch today which gives me instant longitude. It also reminds me of their courageous endeavours.

The sun rises, the sun sets, the moon rises, the moon sets, the Earth spins, the Earth has day, and the Earth has night (Figure 13.2). Our sun, our moon and our Earth's rotation give us our cyclical pattern of life. They give us the light–dark cycle. We are tied to this cycle; it gives our master clock its cues and from this, *our master clock sets our time*.

SYNCHRONY: WHO SETS THE RHYTHM?

When the master clock has set the time, your *master clock sets the rhythm*. Your master clock resets all your body clocks; every single one of your 30 trillion, every day of your life. This ensures that your clocks chime in *synchrony* and things happen in an orderly fashion: you wake, you rise, you go to the loo, you work, you eat, you exercise, you rest, you sleep, you wake... and so it continues. Your body clocks and genes coordinate the hormonal, chemical and genetic responses for each and every action (Figure 13.3).

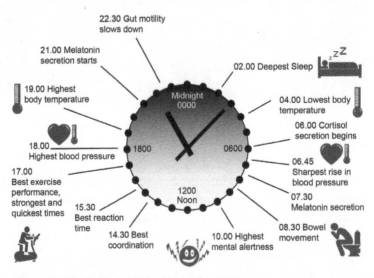

Figure 13.3. The timing of circadian biological processes.

DYSSYNCHRONY: WHERE DID THE RHYTHM GO?

Every day, you set your master clock by daylight, and you set your body clocks by your food (*food what*), food timing (*food when*) and exercise. Under the stewardship of the master clock, all your clocks chime together, and you are in perfect harmony.

But if your body clocks don't get the right cues, or receive conflicting cues, they go out of sync. If a meal is eaten in the middle of the night, the master says 'night', your liver organ clock says 'day', and the clocks stop chiming in sync. This is clock *dyssynchrony*. As your body clocks no longer chime together, your biological processes don't happen quickly or easily, and they don't happen in the right order.

We are all vulnerable to disruption of our body clocks and our circadian rhythm. It only takes one poor night's sleep, an overnight flight, or stress to throw your circadian rhythm into a muddle. Your clocks are much easier to disturb than you may imagine.

The great news is that attention to the two big boys, *daylight* and *food timing*, are huge steps in achieving and maintaining a healthy circadian rhythm.

Dyssynchrony of body clocks is typified by jet lag, social jet lag and shift working. It is a common feature in many long-term metabolic conditions such as insulin resistance, obesity, hypertension and diabetes (see below).

Jet lag

The master clock and body clocks can cope with a maximum change of one hour per day, but no more. Jet lag occurs when you both change the light–dark cycle and alter your food timing by more than one hour a day. Neither your master clock nor your body clocks are synced to the new light–dark cycle, but all the clocks do eventually settle into the new time zone but, scarily for long-haul holidaymakers, it takes one day to recover from each time zone crossed – and then you have to do it again on the return leg!

Social jet lag

Imagine a weekend where you are out both Saturday and Sunday night, eating and drinking late; you sleep until lunchtime both days. When you then have to wake up at your usual time on Monday morning, you will unsurprisingly have the blues. Your metabolism is awry: your sleep hormones don't know if it is night or day. Your Monday wake-up call from your cortisol has gone AWOL and you are not ready for the day. You are not alert and it's difficult to concentrate. It's called social jet lag. You have upset your circadian rhythm and caused body clock dyssynchrony. And that's why you don't like Mondays!

Shift work

Shift workers' light–dark cycle is altered; the act of working all night tells the body clocks that it is daytime, but their master clock is in the dark and signals that it is night. Their clocks are dyssynchronous. With this as well as constantly changing eating patterns and insufficient sleep, their metabolism goes haywire, and metabolic diseases and obesity soon follow.[16] Shift workers have a significantly higher risk of obesity, cancer, diabetes, hypertension, infections and other diseases.[17] The finger points firmly to dyssynchronous body clocks and disturbances of circadian rhythm as the likely cause.[18,19,20] Some people pay a heavy price to keep the wheels of industry turning. If we introduced shift working today, it would carry a health warning.

Long-term circadian disruption and clock dyssynchrony lead to insulin resistance, which is the 'sun' at the centre of our 'metabolic universe' and the first stop on board the metabolic bus to Armageddon. (Figure 1.1) Your lifestyle sets your clocks.

WHAT CHRONOTYPE ARE YOU?

Which is your preferred song? That of the lark at sunrise, or the nocturnal call of the female tawny owl 'too-wit' and the male 'too-woo' reply? Are you a morning lark or a night owl?

Morning larks, who prefer early-to-rise and early-to-bed, outnumber the night owls, who like the opposite. This has made larks the bullies of the sleep world, robbing the night owls of precious and nourishing early morning REM sleep, essential for memory. The world is geared to the tune of the morning lark and cruel to night owls, requiring them to conform to school and work times that don't suit them. Unless they are very careful, they will suffer a life of prolonged sleep deprivation, with all its health consequences.

These distinctive types of sleep patterns are called *morning* and *night chronotypes*. There is a spectrum of chronotypes, with many people in the middle. Your chronotype does change throughout life, thankfully for teenagers! And you can with effort adjust your chronotype to conform to society. Genetic changes have been described that can identify larks or owls, and research continues to evaluate whether certain chronotypes have enhanced risks of metabolic disease.[21,22]

CIRCADIAN RHYTHM AND SLEEP

Sleep is the beginning of our biological day, and one of our most important circadian rhythms. We need to sleep a minimum of seven hours a night and serious health problems may develop if we have six hours' sleep or less. During sleep, vital processes such as repair, regeneration, growth and consolidation of memory are carried out. Lack of sleep is strongly associated with obesity. Loss of sleep for even one night increases insulin resistance.[23,24,25,26,27] We saw in Chapter 10 that we must reverse insulin resistance to lose weight. We now know that sleep is another part of that process.

The process of going to sleep and waking up has a circadian rhythm, and to sleep well your clocks need to be in synchrony. Clock synchrony ensures an appropriate timing of the release and peak of melatonin, which allows you to drift off to sleep quickly (Figure 13.4). Waking up requires the coordination of cortisol release and all the other hormones, to increase your heart rate, your body temperature and your blood pressure, ready for the day.

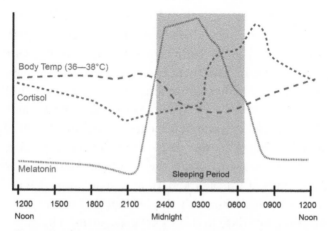

Figure 13.4. Diurnal changes in melatonin, cortisol and body temperature.[57]

CIRCADIAN RHYTHM AND METABOLISM

Metabolism is a term for all the chemical processes in your body that keep you alive. Cells are constantly carrying out thousands of chemical reactions. Metabolism is the foundation of everything that we do; it means breaking down food and drink for energy, and using this energy to support, build and repair your body. It is differences in energy metabolism that make you thin or fat. In turn your metabolism is coordinated by your circadian rhythm.

It is controlled by the master clocks, organ clocks and cell clocks. Your metabolism has a *diurnal pattern*, an innate rhythm corresponding to the Earth day, and is *fine-tuned* by the *timing of light and food*.

The hormones insulin, cortisol and growth hormone are the big guns in metabolism, and they all show rhythmical diurnal patterns, influencing our metabolism so that it responds to the varying demands of our day (Figure 13.4). The rhythm of these and other hormones explains our maximum alertness mid-morning, our peak athletic performances in the afternoon, and increased fat storage at night after a meal, compared to eating an identical meal during the day.

When Eliud Kipchoge, the world's finest marathon runner, became the first person in history to break the two-hour marathon, which he did by 20 seconds, it was a landmark in human performance. The blistering pace was achieved with the help of meticulous planning and support from the INEOS 1:59 challenge team. The time trial took place in the early morning, in a misty park in Vienna. Might the result have been more spectacular if the race had been mid-afternoon, when circadian rhythm indicates maximal performance?

The circadian rhythm of insulin

Insulin is released from the pancreas in a circadian rhythmical pattern.[28,29,30] Rhythm is innate to the pancreatic islet cells (see Chapter 10) that have clocks and follow a 24-hour cycle. Not only do the cells show an innate rhythm, but they can be influenced by the usual suspects, such as melatonin. It may be hard to believe that a dish of cells has rhythm, but this just shows the magic of the *rhythm of life!* And this rhythm of islet pancreatic cells is not confined to the laboratory but has also been confirmed in the living pancreas.[31] A circadian rhythm of insulin affects our handling of meals, our energy storage and thus our waistlines.[32,33]

Not only is the *release* of insulin rhythmical, but its *effect* is too. Insulin sensitivity decreases throughout the day. The flip side is that *insulin resistance increases as the day progresses*. The *later* that a meal is eaten, the *more* insulin is needed.

Insulin resistance, the first step to metabolic disease, is also the key to weight loss and metabolic health. Late-night eating, because it increases insulin resistance, will not help your weight loss; furthermore, late-night eating alone may cause you to gain weight.[34,35,36,37,38,39] The old saying 'breakfast like a king, lunch like a prince and supper like a pauper' now has science behind it. (See Chapter 14, 'Food Timing').

The circadian rhythm of cortisol

As much as you may be excited about every new morning, you need some help to wake up and to face the day. And that's what cortisol does; gives you a boost to start the day. Cortisol levels peak in the morning: this makes you alert, your body temperature goes up, your blood pressure rises, as does your heart rate (Figure 13.4). Once you are up and about, cortisol then returns to its basal level. Your cortisol boost is primed by your circadian rhythm and when you disturb your rhythm, for example when you are jet-lagged, you miss that morning cortisol, you struggle to wake up and when you do, you feel very sluggish, low in energy, moody, with reduced mental function, and everything else that comes with jet lag.[40]

Stress causes persistently elevated cortisol, with loss of the normal diurnal rhythm. This lack of the early morning boost badly affects your sleep, which in turn badly affects your metabolism. Energy storage goes awry, and this is followed by weight gain. Thus, managing stress is critical for weight loss.[41] Managing stress well means that the elevated levels of cortisol disappear, it returns to its normal circadian rhythm, your metabolism recovers and weight reduces.

The circadian rhythm of growth hormone

Growth hormone has a diurnal rhythm and its levels peak when you are asleep. This allows all the body's routine cleaning and maintenance to be carried out at night, so that you can do the big glory things during the day. High levels of growth hormone switch the appropriate genes on and off to allow this maintenance to be carried out.

If you don't sleep well, then your maintenance regime suffers and you age badly. Poor sleep caused by clock dyssynchrony has adverse effects on your metabolism, your immune system and your brain function.

CIRCADIAN RHYTHM: OBESITY AND FOOD

Obesity

When your circadian rhythm sings, you sing. You sleep well, you are lean and healthy. Synchronous clocks control your body's natural processes. Digestion and sleep happen at different times, with hormones being produced to cope with digestion or sleep, but not both at the same time. Ever gone to bed late at night, having just eaten a big meal, and found yourself unable to sleep? Now you have the answer: dyssynchronous clocks.

What happens if you get up in the middle of the night and eat? Gut bugs are asleep, no enzymes are ready, sphincters are all contracted (thankfully), and the genetic machinery of digestion is switched off. Sensing an onslaught, emergency digestion, absorption and storage switch on. Late-night 'goodies' are sent straight to the fat stores. Nowhere else wants or needs them. And that's why snacking during the night is a behaviour associated with obesity.

Food *type*, food *timing* and food *frequency* all reset the organs' clocks, but this goes under the radar of the master clock, which responds mainly to light. Food timing is the ultimate disruptor to clock synchrony. As well as keeping your EatSpan to under 10 hours, this part of the obesity puzzle is really that simple.

Food timing

Digestion, absorption and energy storage is also a huge set of co-ordinated actions, involving hormones, gut bugs, gut movement and enzymes, to name but a few of the players. Like in an orchestra, rhythm and timing are the keys to success.[42]

Eating all day

Food processing is an immensely complicated process, requiring hundreds of genes switching on and off. It starts even before your first mouthful, when a *cephalic release* of insulin primes your gut for action. Digestive juices are prepared, even just by thinking about food. You may have noticed a spurt of saliva from your mouth at the sight or thought of food! Genes are turned on and enzymes are made, stomach acid increases ready to repel invaders, gut motility increases and food is propelled down the gut. Gene activation alters and changes the gut lining, so nutrients cross the gut wall, at platform 9¾ (see Chapter 3). In the liver, packing systems are primed, food is processed, exported via carriers, and the liver sends nutrients to the storage depots. Genes are turned off and the hunger hormone ghrelin disappears. Genes to make the satiety hormone leptin are turned on. Insulin patrols the bloodstream, searching for keyholes to open storage doors, allowing fat and sugars to flow into fat cells and muscles.

This entire cycle of food processing can take up to four hours at the best of times. Late at night – the worst of times – it can take much longer. The body, while a masterpiece of design, cannot keep the food processing system up for ever. The liver cannot perform 24/7; we must give it a rest, from food as well as booze. At most, the digestive system works well for 8–10 hours per day. A lifestyle where you force your body to cope with food over longer periods means the metabolic bus!

A recognised feature of modern life is the trend away from set meals to a pattern of grazing throughout the day.[43] The clock starts ticking with the first bite of the day, which resets the organ clocks. If you eat all day, the organ clocks receive food timing messages that reset their clocks and, working alone, under the radar of the master clock, clock dyssynchrony occurs.[44]

To live in harmony with your body clocks, food timing messages to the organ clocks must coincide with light messages, which feed into the master clock. And this means eating within an 8–10-hour EatSpan window, with a 14–16 FastSpan.[45,46,47] Of course it matters *what* food you eat, but it also matters *when* you eat. In other words, *what food*, *when food* and *food frequency*.

Late-night eating

As insulin resistance increases with late-night eating, it makes perfect sense to avoid those late-night snacks, but that's a hard ask for many people. Eating at night resets the digestive organ clocks, and dyssynchrony plays havoc with your digestion and circadian rhythm. The master clock is expecting the cleaners, not the digestors; it doesn't expect you to eat just before you go to bed.

Late-night eating can take the form of two patterns. It is usually described as eating after six p.m. or within two hours of bedtime. Both these patterns of eating are associated with increased insulin resistance, metabolic abnormalities and obesity. In an ideal world, your last meal at night should be finished by six p.m. And that includes drinks.

This timing may just not fit in with modern life and a reasonable compromise is to aim to finish eating 3–4 hours before bedtime. Two hours before bedtime is the *critical time* and ideally, to avoid clock dyssynchrony, nothing should be eaten or drunk during this time. Water excepted of course.

Meal routine

We are rhythmical creatures, and we sway to the beat of our body clocks. Repeated changes in meal routines require the organ clocks to continually reset. Irregular mealtimes cause clock dyssynchrony, but regular mealtimes mean synchronous body clocks and health.[48] This is therefore a laudable aim.

CHRONO-NUTRITION

There are places in the world that we have looked at briefly already, where people live a long time and are well for most of their lives. Rather than boarding the metabolic bus, they forge their own path, and usually by foot. They don't get metabolic diseases, nor are they obese, remaining healthy until late in life. Called the Blue Zones, these corners of the planet have the highest number of centenarians in the world (Figure 13.5).

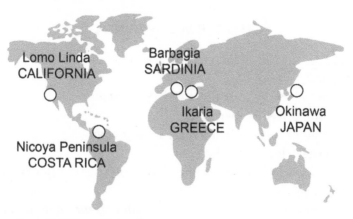

Figure 13.5. The world's Blue Zones.

Some of the features of their lives are what you would probably expect: they do not eat processed foods; they eat a healthy diet, rich in plants and with lots of fat, which fits the description of the Mediterranean diet. But also, people in the Blue Zones *eat little or nothing in the evening.*[49,50] The smallest meal of the day is eaten last, in the afternoon or early evening, and nothing is eaten after that. So not only do they have a long FastSpan, about 14–16 hours, but also the amount and timing of their meals fits in with the natural rhythms of life.

This is what chrono-nutrition is all about: synchronising your body clocks to your master clock. Chrono-nutrition means that the food messages going to your body clocks are in sync with the light messages going to your master clock.

> *As earthlings, we are tied to the light–dark cycle of our beautiful and fragile planet.*

Chrono-nutrition looks at using the timing and composition of nutrition to reverse both obesity and disease.[51,52,53,54] As a science it is still evolving and while much is known, there are still many unknown knowns and unknown unknowns.[55,56] Your *12-week reset plan* has its roots in the field of chrono-nutrition. We've taken the known knowns and used these principles to create it. As with any science, findings will surely emerge to add to our well-founded beliefs, and your new-found knowledge.

CHAPTER WHISPERINGS

- Circadian rhythm is the control and ordering of your biological processes.
- A master clock in your brain sets the time.
- Every organ has its own clock.
- Every one of your 30 trillion cells has a clock.
- The master clock is set by light.
- The master clock controls the timing of your body clocks and resets them daily.
- The master clock sets the circadian rhythm to the light–dark cycle, to which we are tied.
- The master clock responds to blue light messages relayed from the eye. Light is interpreted as daytime and an absence of light is interpreted as night time.
- Your body clocks have an innate rhythm.
- The strongest external influencers (zeitgebers) are light, food timing and exercise.
- Clocks work in synchrony with the master clock in good health.
- Most biological processes have a circadian rhythm.
- Dyssynchronous clocks are associated with insulin resistance, abnormal metabolism, obesity, diabetes and other metabolic diseases.
- Jet lag, social jet lag and shift working are all associated with clock dyssynchrony.
- Different chronotypes – night owls and morning larks – have different sleep preferences and genetic signatures.
- Sleep deprivation both causes, and results from, clock dyssynchrony.
- Knowing about circadian rhythm teaches you when to turn out the lights and chrono-nutrition is the science of eating in tune with all your body clocks.

PART THREE

THE WHISPERER PLANS

THE WHISPERER PLANS

12-Week Plan, en route to weight loss and wellness

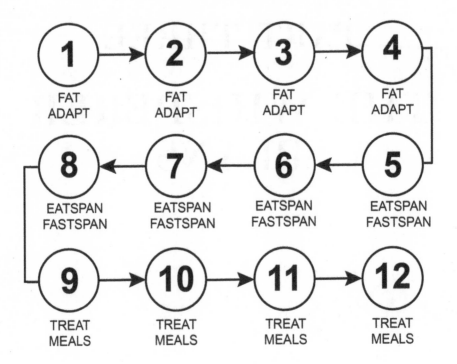

14

THE DIET WHISPERER
SECRETS

Nor is it wiser to weep a true occasion lost, but trim
our sails, and let old bygones be.

Alfred Lord Tennyson (1809–92)

There are three plans for your whisperer journey, so you can choose
the one that suits you best. They are:

1. The Diet Whisperer 12-week reset plan for fat loss: *whisperer-loss*.
2. The Diet Whisperer plan to keep you at your target weight:
   whisperer-stable.
3. The Diet Whisperer plan for times in the future should your weight
   increase: *whisperer-recover*.

You will begin with the 12-week *whisperer-loss plan*. It is reasonable to expect weight loss of 1–2 pounds (0.5–1.0 kg) per week,
depending on your size. If you have more than 26 pounds (12 kg)
to lose, complete the 12-week plan, then go back and repeat weeks
9–12. Continue this four-week cycle, and keep repeating this four-
week plan, until you achieve your target weight.

Once you have achieved your target weight, move on to the
whisperer-stable plan. This provides you with a stable weight and
excellent metabolism henceforth. Should you subsequently err, and
put on a few pounds, adopt the *whisperer-recover plan*. This will
rapidly get you back to where you want to be.

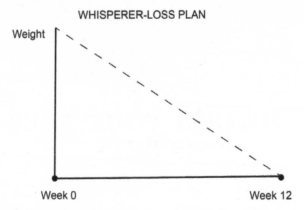

WHISPERER-LOSS PLAN

Figure 14.1. The whisperer-loss plan.

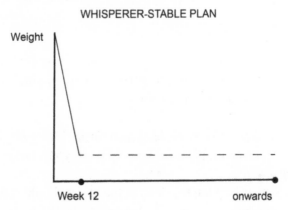

WHISPERER-STABLE PLAN

Figure 14.2. The whisperer-stable plan.

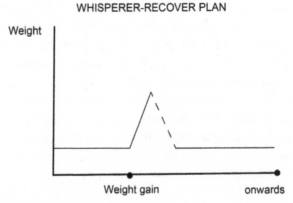

WHISPERER-RECOVER PLAN

Figure 14.3. The whisperer-recover plan.

When you finish the *whisperer-loss plan*, you will have found the secrets to permanent weight loss. You will have the tools to lose weight, to maintain a steady weight and to correct any future indiscretions. You will be in control of your weight. And you will be able to help your family and friends. You will be a *diet whisperer*.

WHISPERER FUNDAMENTALS

1. *Fat adaptation*, relearning to burn fat for fuel.
2. *No snacking*, providing periods without.
3. *Reduce EatSpan* and *increase FastSpan* every day.
4. *Remove* quickly digested (super-refined and refined) carbs from your diet.
5. *Lifestyle management changes* support your whisperer journey; reduce stress, sleep more than seven hours a night, respecting your natural rhythms, and share a positive social circle with family and friends.

WHISPERER FOOD

1. *Eat real food.* You should eat high-quality food, preferably organic, and avoid processed food at all costs.
2. *Super-refined carbohydrates* and processed foods contain high sugar levels and multiple additives: sugar, bad fats, preservatives, colourings and other toxic chemicals. Playing havoc with your hormones, these foods are not part of your 12-week plan.
3. *Refined carbohydrates* will also upset your hormones and prevent weight loss, and these need to be avoided for the duration of the 12-week plan, other than as part of your treat meals.
4. *Adequate intake of healthy PUFA omega-3s, and lower omega-6s. Get the omega-6/3 ratio correct,* to reduce systemic inflammation.
5. *Avoid foods labelled as low-fat;* these foods often contain sugar and/or high fructose corn syrup.
6. *The whisperer plan is a low-carb, high-fat diet,* used as a springboard into fat adaptation.
7. Removing good fats from your diet is associated with weight gain and fat fuel inhibition.

WHISPERER FOOD TIMING

1. The shorter the EatSpan and the longer the FastSpan, the greater the fat burning.
2. Aim for an EatSpan of less than 10 hours.
3. You should eat a maximum of three meals per day – and every snack counts as a meal.
4. Once you introduce intermittent fasting, at week 5, the number of meals reduces.
5. The earlier you eat your meals, the more this fits in with natural rhythms (see Chapter 13). Eating a greater proportion of your food earlier in the day, even if the amount is kept the same, results in less insulin release. Our plans from week 5 are based around lunch and supper. You may prefer plans based around breakfast or lunch. The plans are flexible enough, and your knowledge at this stage good enough, to decide for yourself.
6. For the 'two-meal days', as a rule of thumb, for your long-term health and weight control breakfast and lunch are *marginally* better than lunch and supper. This means FastSpan is extended either before or after your night's sleep. We personally find it easier to extend in the morning, particularly for beginners and those working. Don't do breakfast and supper; this really messes up your EatSpan and FastSpan.

WHISPERER RULES

Record your food data

A food diary is important for success, and you can use your weight loss journal or an online food diary. We suggest that every day, you record the number of meals, your EatSpan and FastSpan and the macro composition of each meal.

Enter your personalised macros from the keto calculator on the website, enter your daily foods, and then you can track progress. We perfectly understand that some people find it too time-consuming or stressful to do this, but at the very least try it for the first two or three weeks. In the beginning, too, tracking will help you with portion sizes.

Compare your successes with your group and if you fail to meet your goals on day 1, or 4, or 24, put it behind you and get back to concentrating on the day at hand. Look back at your data and count your success days and stay positive. The whisperer encourages you to record the number of meals, EatSpan and FastSpan, and total these each week. You will be amazed to see the number of meals reduce as the plan progresses!

No snacking

It is critical that you do not ever snack between meals. If you have a really tough carb withdrawal, you can have some 'rescue apples', but they reduce over the first three weeks. It is equally critical that nothing is taken between your last meal and getting up in the morning (FastSpan). What is permitted is water, black coffee or black tea. You may want to consider decaffeinated tea and coffee, if you are taking drinks around bedtime.

Exercise

a) *not doing cardio:* If you normally live a sedentary life, do not start an exercise programme now. There will be plenty of time in the future to make exercise part of your life; it is a critical ingredient for good metabolic health, but if you suddenly increase your exercise it will cause your weight loss to stall.

b) *already doing cardio:* then please continue. Your performance will dip, as your body 'fat adapts', but it will recover. If you are an ultra-runner, then running in the fasted state will be part of your endurance fat adaptation. Concentrate on base and avoid tempo and go slow for success later. Watch your zones, as your heart rate will initially be high at the same speed. Go slow for best results later!

c) *not doing resistance training:* Just imagine, you are trying to lose weight, all your hormones are pointing towards catabolism and fat burning, and you try to change direction to anabolism and muscle building. Your body is a miracle worker, but it cannot burn fat *and* build muscle at the same time. So, until you have reached your target weight, if you don't normally do resistance training, don't start now.

d) *already doing resistance training:* then please continue. Studies have shown that if training is maintained, you will maintain lean tissue as you lose weight. However, it's best to forget about building muscle. The aim of your 12 weeks is to maintain your lean tissue and your resistance programme should change from one of building to one of maintenance. If you take protein shakes outside mealtimes, they will have to go for now; they will play havoc with your hormones and stimulate an insulin response, which will stop fat burning, and this will stop weight loss. The diet has a moderate protein content, which will be enough to preserve your lean body mass. If you are desperate, give up the protein shakes for the first four weeks and then if you must reintroduce them, take them at mealtimes. We'd rather you got to your target weight first.

Alcohol

We advise against alcohol for the duration of the 12-week plan. It inhibits fat burning, as your liver is busy detoxifying the alcohol.

If you are someone who simply cannot give up alcohol, you can still benefit hugely from the 12-week plan. Some strategies will help you to succeed, despite continuing to drink alcohol. Do whatever you can in the first four weeks to drink as little as possible; you will be able to return to drinking in time. If you normally drink 'rounds' when socialising, replace your beer with a single measure of spirits; this will reduce your alcohol consumption significantly. A pint of beer contains two units of alcohol, whereas a single shot of gin or vodka contains one unit. Your tolerance to alcohol will be *much* lower than it was. Be very cautious!

The following alcoholic drinks are *relatively* fat adaptation friendly:

1. Vodka with sparkling water and lime with a shot of bitters.
2. Gin (or vodka) and tonic. Any carbs in the tonic form part of your daily carb allowance. Diet tonics have sweeteners that are harmful to your gut bugs, but will be fine for the relatively short period of your 12-week reset plan.
3. Red wine.
4. Champagne.

You'll note that beer is absent from this list; it really is not helpful when trying to burn fat, as it contains too many carbs. To achieve successful weight loss, it must go.

TIPS FOR SUCCESS

Your Partner

One of your best options for success is to involve your partner. It really is very difficult to do any diet alone. Explain to your partner that your metabolic hormonal changes will alter your mood initially, sometimes quite severely. The more your hormones are out of line at the start, the more difficult the first week will be. If you have had a bad diet for a long time and are carb addicted, you will have a degree of 'cold turkey' following your refined carb withdrawal. You may even need to take the first week off work. You will have bad days, difficulty sleeping, bad moods and hunger – but this will all pass (tell your partner this) as your hormones sort themselves out.

Groups

The first four weeks are not going to be easy, but every day is one day closer to being better. If you adopt the plan with your partner, or a group of friends or family, it will be so much easier. You will be able to share your experience, and both give and receive encouragement. Always remember, this plan will change your life for the better. And keep repeating this to yourself. Think of starting a social media group with like-minded friends.

Measurements

Measurements, and recording of these measurements in your weight loss journal, are highly motivational. The most useful measurements are your weight and your waist and hip circumference. Height can also be included for various calculators on the website.

Tools

Spoil yourself and buy a nice set of bathroom scales and weigh in on waking, every day. Empty your bladder, weigh yourself naked and be consistent in the timing. You should buy yourself a tailor's measuring tape. Measure your waist and hips. Both your weight and abdominal girth will go up and down. Be patient, because with time, impressive things will happen.

Treat meals

There is light at the end of the tunnel. In week 9, we will show you how to keep your hormones in order while affording yourself some treat meals, perhaps a curry or your favourite Thai. We will show you how these can be an enjoyable part of a healthy eating plan. However, some people neither need nor want a treat meal and this is perfectly fine too.

THE 12-WEEK RESET PLAN IN REAL LIFE

We have been quite didactic in the plans, but we do understand that in real life you have to meet the demands of work and family. We also know that busy people may not want to get into the calculations; in that case, make sure your net carbs are only 25–50 grams per day and get cracking! We suggest you sit down on a Sunday and plan the week ahead, adapting the plan and choosing your days, especially in week 5 for fasting, and week 9 for treat meals. The plan will have two key factors for you to follow:

Food: Follow a typical ketogenic diet with low carbohydrate, high fat and moderate protein for 12 weeks, except for occasional treat meals, where you can increase the carbs eaten by including refined carbs, but not super-refined carbs.

Food timing: Your EatSpan and FastSpan will be adjusted for optimum fat loss. As the plan progresses, your EatSpan will decrease and your FastSpan will increase. In an ideal world our EatSpan will be 10 hours or less, and our FastSpan 14 hours or more.

15

YOUR PERSONAL GOALS

We are what we repeatedly do. Excellence, then, is not an act, but a habit.

The Story of Philosophy, Will Durant, 1926

Changing to a new diet and lifestyle is hard for everyone and you may struggle to believe in yourself. You have probably followed many different diets and your confidence may be low. People have told us on countless occasions that they have lost weight in the past, only to find that they just put it all back on again; but this all changed when they found the whisperer plan. The *12-week reset plan* not only allows you to lose weight and regain your health, but gives you the tools to keep the weight off for ever and stay healthy.

You may feel success is impossible, but don't worry: relax, sit back, and get ready to embark on your 12-week plan. We will guide you through the potential pitfalls and help you to emerge victorious.

We all know that motivation can wax and wane, so we will help you to stay motivated throughout the plan with useful tips and guidance. You should follow each of the following points to help you with your weight loss journey; your path to a healthy metabolism and a new-look you.

If you want to succeed, you need to set goals. This is a proven way of increasing your chance of successful permanent weight loss; so even if you are sceptical, we urge you to do it.[1,2,3,4] You can also use your goals in times of struggle. Like us, everyone struggles at some point, and it is naïve to think otherwise.

DETERMINE YOUR GOALS

You should use the things that motivate you to set your goals, and everyone's motivation is different. You can have several goals, but not too many, as this may complicate your journey. Two or three are usually sufficient.

Weight loss is likely to be your primary goal, but there are other goals you may consider. Common goals are reducing waist circumference, or improving waist-to-hip ratio (see Chapter 8).

Your goals should be a specific task, for a defined length of time; 'I want to lose twelve pounds in twelve weeks' is a good goal, compared to a statement such as 'I want to lose weight soon.' The latter is less likely to motivate you and so you are less likely to succeed.

You should be able to measure your goal; for example you may want to reduce your belly size (a good goal, as this correlates with good metabolic health). You could select your waist–hip ratio as a measurable outcome; measure waist and hips regularly, and chart your progress.

Your goal will need to be attainable; we find that a maximum of 26 pounds (12 kg) weight loss for the 12 weeks is safe and achievable. You can lose as much weight as you like on the whisperer plan by repeating weeks 9–12 as often as is required. You can choose 26 pounds in 12 weeks and at the end, make a new goal and extend your journey with a new time frame (Figure 15.1).

We can't stress enough that you need to set your own goals; this will drive your motivation throughout your whisperer journey. And only you know what motivates you! Setting your own goals is so much more powerful than if someone else such as ourselves or your doctor sets them for you.

Once you set your goals, you will need to write them down. This is the most powerful way to attain them. Looking at goals in black and white makes them real, makes them tangible and more achievable. Make sure that your goals are positive and come from within, reflecting your true desires.

STRONG GOALS	vs	WEAK GOALS
1. I will lose 20 pounds in 20 days		1. I want to lose weight soon
2. I will drop 2 inches from my waist in 12 weeks		2. I want to look better
3. I will reduce my blood pressure to 120/80 in 12 weeks		3. I want to improve my metabolism
4. I will be able to fast for 24 hours within 12 weeks		4. I want to learn to fat adapt
5. I will sleep for a minimum of 7 hours every night within 4 weeks		5. I'd like to sleep better
6. I will go to bed at 10.00 pm every night from Monday		6. I'm going to improve my sleep routine
7. I will begin a meditation course by the end of the month		7. I need to de-stress soon
8. I will eat over 30 grams of fibre every day from Monday		8. I need to eat more vegatables

Figure 15.1. Examples of strong and weak goals.

WEIGHT LOSS JOURNAL

A weight loss journal is a proven way to increase your chances of weight loss and your success may well depend on this. It may seem a bit quaint to manually record your progress in a journal, but scores of testimonials, studies and data prove the benefits of doing so. You can find weight loss journals online, or in bookshops, in both digital and analogue form. We have a weight loss journal on our website.

Tracking your food intake means that you are more likely to lose weight. With your low-carb, high-fat diet in the *12-week reset plan*, you will need to know the composition of your daily diet so you can ensure that you maintain the correct proportion of macronutrients.

As your weight loss journal develops, it will provide you with a description of your unique journey, your goals, your coping strategies, your strengths and your weaknesses. It may also teach you a lot about your drivers. Record your goals, your successes and your failures and watch as you develop and change on your journey (Figure 15.2).

SHARE YOUR GOALS

Sharing your goals is going to help you a lot. You will quickly find out who supports you and who doesn't. There will be lots of people in your tribe who support you and wish you well – they may even join you – so focus on these people. Avoid negative people and negative comments.

When you share your goals, you are giving power to them and making them a reality. If you make a public commitment, you are much more likely to achieve your goals.

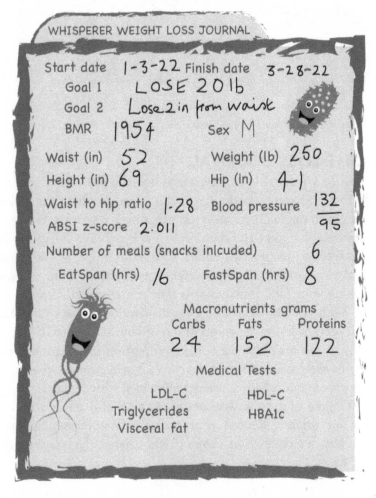

WHISPERER WEIGHT LOSS JOURNAL

Start date 1-3-22 Finish date 3-28-22
    Goal 1   LOSE 20 lb
    Goal 2   Lose 2 in from waist
    BMR 1954   Sex M

Waist (in) 52   Weight (lb) 250
Height (in) 69   Hip (in) 41

Waist to hip ratio 1·28   Blood pressure 132/95
ABSI z-score 2.011

Number of meals (snacks inlcuded)   6

    EatSpan (hrs) 16   FastSpan (hrs) 8

                    Macronutrients grams
            Carbs   Fats   Proteins
            24   152   122
                    Medical Tests
            LDL-C   HDL-C
        Triglycerides   HBA1c
        Visceral fat

Figure 15.2. Goals and metrics in a male weighing 250 lb. Medical test results are optional.

FAILURE

The fact is, we aren't always successful. Life gets in the way, our motivation drops, temptation proves too much and everything in our plan disintegrates. But failure can bring success; sometimes you fail a number of times before you succeed.

If you go off-piste unintentionally, don't give up. Dust yourself down and start again; make each day your masterpiece. Your resolve to succeed will be strengthened by your failure and you will be more resolute. Remember the saying 'To err is human, to forgive divine'. Find the capacity to forgive yourself and carry on with your plan.

You might like to have a strategy for failure, so if something happens you will be prepared for it. For example, you are invited to an important social event, you probably will not be able to follow the diet, and you don't want to ruin everyone else's fun. Just accept that for that day, you are having a treat and the following day you will regroup.

Or just accept that on Sunday (say), you ate too much food, you ate food that was on the banned list, and you enjoyed it! But make this a one-off; on Monday, resume your weight loss journey. Don't beat yourself up, don't be self-defeating and pitying, just carry on with your weight loss journey. You don't have to be perfect to lose weight.

Triggers

If you are an emotional or a comfort eater, you probably respond to stress or other intense emotions by snacking, and snacks are not part of your 12-week plan. If you can identify your triggers, you will be able to plan a strategy to deal with them. Everyone is different and everyone has their own trigger. It may be boredom, or a reward for positive or negative emotions. Recognising your triggers is the first powerful step in changing this behaviour pattern.

Once you have identified your trigger(s), it's time to plan alternative reactions to them and quit the snacking. Let's say anxiety is a trigger. When you are challenged, you react by eating a biscuit. Now you need to make a plan that when you are next challenged, you do not eat a biscuit, you now react in a different way. Perhaps you go for a stroll, or go somewhere quiet and take deep breaths; anything to head off your usual reaction. You will have managed your stress in a way that no longer involves food, and your weight loss plan will stay on track.

YOUR ACTION PLAN

Once you have set your goals, you need to create an action plan. You should follow the whisperer general principles, identified in the previous chapter. You will need to see how these principles fit in with your lifestyle and juggle it around so that it works for you.

The first thing to do is to identify when you are going to start your 12-week plan. Try to find a period in the near future when your commitments are minimal, you have no great demands on your time and your normal social support is intact; when you can see that you will have the strength to devote most of your energy to your weight loss journey.

Once you have identified the 'when', put your date in your weight loss journal and let your friends and family know. You will need to plan how your food plan fits in with your family and work out the logistics. If you regularly eat out or have takeaways, this will need to change. You will need to work out how to shop for food and prepare your meals instead.

If you are on medication or have a long-term disease, you will need to seek the advice of your doctor before embarking on your plan. You may wish to have blood tests or other investigations such as visceral fat measurements before you start on the plan; they will be useful for comparisons once you have finished.

CHAPTER WHISPERINGS

- A new diet and lifestyle are challenging for everyone.
- Motivation is the key to achieving your desired weight loss.
- Setting goals will increase your motivation and help with your whisperer journey.
- Your goals should be time-limited, positive, measurable and achievable.

- Writing down your goals in a weight loss journal will help you to be more successful.
- Share your goals with your family and friends.
- Plan for the odd blip; from this will come success.
- Before you start, if you are taking medication or have any long-term diseases you should see your doctor.

16

THE 12-WEEK RESET PLAN: FOOD

There is no love sincerer than the love of food.
Man and Superman, George Bernard Shaw, 1903

The key to weight loss is to learn to use your fat stores to supply energy in your body. This means relearning to use your fat-burning engine by fat adaptation (see Chapter 11).

In your *12-week reset plan*, to achieve fat adaptation you will eat a low-carbohydrate, high-fat diet with moderate protein content. This is a keto or ketogenic diet, which we use as a springboard into *fat adaptation*. Your body's cells will burn fat as their primary fuel, and as your brain cannot do this, it feeds off the ketone bodies, which help it cleanse and detox.

Fat adaptation will take some time, as these pathways will be a little rusty, and it will take practice for your body to make them as efficient as your carb pathways. However, fuelling with fat is a perfectly natural state and once you're fat adapted, you will be able to use fat to fuel with impunity. Remember, although your body is designed to survive quite happily on ketones, it may take a bit of persuasion.

TIPS FOR YOUR 12-WEEK RESET PLAN

KETO FLU
Everyone deals with a low-carb, high-fat diet differently and it is not uncommon to have problems in the early stages of switching from a

carb-burning engine to a fat-burning engine. The more dependent you are on carbs; the more sluggish your switch and greater the likelihood of keto flu. If you are already fat adapted, your switch will be much easier.

Keto flu is not a viral infection but a response to the withdrawal of carbs, and develops in the first week after dietary change. Not everyone develops keto flu, but for those who do, the symptoms can be unpleasant.[1,2] (Figure 16.1.)

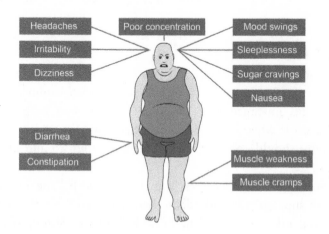

Figure 16.1. Metabolic Man with 'keto flu'.

The good news is that keto flu will resolve. The symptoms will lessen and disappear; this can take a week, but sometimes longer, even up to a month, depending on your metabolism when you started. A very small number of people will not settle but this is unusual.

How to Prevent and Manage Keto Flu

Introducing the low-carb diet slowly will help to minimise keto flu. Firstly, withdraw all super-refined carbs; then, if you are well, introduce the full low-carb, high-fat diet. If, after the first week, you are really struggling with keto flu, you can repeat the first week.

It is very important to ensure that you are properly hydrated. The recommended daily allowance is three litres of water for men and 2.3 litres for women.[3] Your water intake can be covered by other fluids: green or unsweetened herbal tea or black coffee. Your fluids should be increased if you live in a hot environment, or you are physically active.

Drinking fluids throughout the day is helpful and thirst is a reliable indicator of dehydration. If you do not feel thirsty and your urine is consistently light yellow or colourless, then you are probably drinking enough.

Ensure that the timing of your plan is during a relatively quiet time of your life. We have already discussed involving your loved ones in your plan, and it is important that they support you in your quest for weight loss and health. You will need to ask for their forbearance, as you may not quite be yourself during these first few weeks.

DO NOT HIT THE GYM

Once you start your 12-week plan you need to be kind to yourself; now is not the time to embark on an exercise programme. Do not under any circumstances 'hit the gym' now. If you wish to start exercising, do it when you reach your target weight. If you already exercise, you should continue as before, but avoid a build phase of training.

You should get plenty of rest and lots of sleep. The internet is awash with supplements and pills to help you with keto flu, but you should avoid taking these. Your body has all the resources that it needs to make the transition; just be patient until it has set up the necessary pathways to work effortlessly and smoothly and fat adapt.

IS A LOW-CARB DIET SAFE?

A low-carb, high-fat diet is safe in the short term and safe for your 12-week plan (but see contraindications below). Your body needs fat and protein and can happily live without carbs, and problems are rare.[4,5] Keto diets are used medically for several conditions including childhood epilepsy.[6]

It can be quite hard to eat enough fibre on a low-carb diet, so you need to plan to maximise your fibre and use your carb allowance for the all-important green vegetables.

And like any restrictive diet, a low-carb, high-fat diet does have potential problems, if followed in the long term. We will not ask you to follow a keto diet for longer than it takes to achieve your target weight, during which it is perfectly safe.[7,8] This short-term restriction will have huge long-term benefits. Once you reach your desired weight and move to the *whisperer-stable plan*, you will be able to increase your dietary fibre. The dietary emphasis will then be feeding your gut bugs, eating a wide variety of real foods and avoiding chemicals.

Potential side effects include gout, fat deposition in the liver, change in blood fat profile, and kidney stones. Long-term restrictive diets have also been associated with nutritional deficiencies, but these are unlikely to occur in the *whisperer-loss* time frame. If you develop any new or unexplained symptoms while on this diet, you should see your doctor.

HIGH QUALITY VERSUS LOW QUALITY FOOD

The principles of your diet are to maintain a low carb intake and a high fat intake. But the type of fats and carbs that you eat is important. At one end of the spectrum, we have processed food, and at the other end, real organic whole food.

You may think that tinkering with fast food to avoid carbs will do the trick. For example eating a double cheeseburger without the bun, or deep-fried chicken without the French fries. But I'm sorry to tell you that this is not the type of food that will help you to lose weight or improve your metabolism. If you eat ultra-processed food, you will have a very high intake of omega-6s, which cause inflammation, a high intake of trans fats, which cause heart disease, and a high intake of preservatives, colourings and pesticides, which will damage your health.[9] Such food is nutrient-poor, deficient in fibre and toxic. It really could not be clearer; if you are going to go to all the effort of improving your metabolism and losing weight, then ultra-processed food will have to go.

Change the burger for a grilled steak and eat with a salad or greens, change the deep-fried chicken for roast chicken! And if you like mint sauce, or gravy, that's fine. But watch out for other sauces (e.g. brown, red and chilli sauce), which may be laced with sugar and fructose. With healthy fats, nutritious food and plenty of fibre you will be on the road to weight loss and health (Figure 16.2).

ARTIFICIAL SWEETENERS

Fizzy drinks are a major cause of metabolic problems and obesity. We wince when we see children with two-litre bottles of 'full sugar pop', thinking of their livers and insulin resistance building.[10] They don't understand what is happening to their fragile metabolism, as they develop fizzy drink syndrome (see Chapter 4), but you do! As people became wise to this, the appetite for sweetened fizzy drinks waned; but undaunted, the corporates introduced diet versions, marketed as an alternative to metabolic Armageddon. We are now being conned into thinking that drinking diet fizzy drinks is healthy and safe, but this is not true.[11] Artificial sweeteners, hailed as the great saviour to our metabolic problems, are not so sweet after all. They are associated with insulin resistance, obesity and an increased chance of developing diabetes.[12,13] The only way to improve your metabolic health and to lose weight is to ditch all fizzy drinks, including the diet versions, for ever. Water is always the winner.

CONTRAINDICATIONS TO THE KETO DIET

A ketogenic diet is contraindicated in patients with disorders of fat metabolism, pancreatitis, carnitine deficiency, carnitine palmitoyl transferase deficiency, carnitine translocase deficiency liver failure, porphyria and pyruvate kinase deficiency. Acetone can be reduced to isopropanol by hepatic alcohol dehydrogenase, which can give a false positive alcohol breath test.[14] Always talk to your doctor before embarking on any restrictive diet, particularly if you have diabetes, hypertension or kidney disease.

UNDERSTANDING KETO DIET NUMBERS

If numbers aren't your thing, and you want to concentrate on one solid rule, then let it be this: **get your net carbs below 25–50 grams per day, and crack on!** The numbers can be confusing, so if you want that perfect plan, stick with me and I'll make it as simple as possible.

1. When we talk about ideal percentages to achieve a state of ketogenesis in the body we are talking about *calories*. The proportions are: carbs 5 per cent, fats 70 per cent and protein 25 per cent. We refer to these figures without any range and without the percentage sign: carbs 5, fats 70 and protein 25. And we use the following abbreviations: carbs = C, fats = F and protein = P. We then put these together to give us the macronutrient type, followed by the percentage of our daily calorie allowance: so C5:F70:P25.

2. To calculate these for yourself, you first need to know your daily

calorie burn or basal metabolic rate (BMR). To calculate your BMR, go the website calculators and enter your details.

3. Record your BMR and enter your BMR into the macronutrient calculator page. This will compute your daily grams of macro-nutrients for your food plan. As you lose weight, repeat and adjust.

4. You will have figures that look something like this: carbs 25 g, fats 156 g and protein 125 g. This represents the weight of the macronutrients, in grams, that make up your *total daily food* for the 12-week plan.

   IMPORTANT: These figures are for *each day*. For each meal divide by three. For the above example this gives us *per meal* carbs 8 g, fats 52 g and protein 42 g. This can be thought of as your *'plate portion'*.

   IMPORTANT: When you go to two meals per day, stick with these numbers or 'plate portion'. DO NOT divide your daily allowance by two. A plate portion is always your daily grams divided by three. The *plate portion* size is the same whether it is one, two or three meals per day. In other words, you don't get three meals in one!

5. Note that macronutrient percentages will be different from calorie percentages. Do not worry about this; it is due to each macro-nutrient having different calories per gram.

   You may be an ounces person. To convert grams to ounces, 100 g = 3.5 ounces, or go to the website for help.

6. Another question we are asked frequently at Whisperer HQ is about 'net carbs'. Net carbs are total carbs minus the fibre. This can be read on any food label.

   Net Carbs = Total Carbs – Fibre

In all our calculations we use *net carbs*. If you eat too many carbs, you will not become ketotic and you will not fat adapt, nor lose weight. So, your carb intake is the most critical.

FOOD LIST

We discussed the principles of food for your 12-week plan in the last chapter. Figure 16.2 now shows you which specific foods to eat and those to avoid.

WHAT TO EAT

Fats and Protein

Fish, shellfish, beef, lamb, pork, poultry, venison and other meats, cream, butter, Greek yoghurt, eggs, and cheeses; brie, cheddar, comte, gruyere, parmesan, feta, halloumi, mascarpone, mozarella, reblochon, vacherin

Fruit

Strawberries, raspberries, blueberries, blackberries

Fresh Vegatables

Leafy greens, spinach, kale, salad greens, lettuce, watercress, herbs, mushrooms, avocado, green beans, runner beans, Brussels sprouts, broccoli, cauliflower, cabbage, celery, asparagus, tomatoes, cucumber, courgettes, green peppers, aubergines, olives, onions, garlic, chillies, potato skins, beansprouts

Oils

Cold-pressed, extra virgin olive oil (EVOO), coconut oil, goose fat, lard, tallow, pork fat, butter and ghee, nut oil, walnut oil, avocado oil

Nuts in increasing carb content

Pecans, Brazil nuts, macadamia nuts, hazelnuts, walnuts, almonds, pine nuts

Seeds Chia, flax, sesame, sunflower

Drinks Black coffee, black tea, green tea, chamomile tea

WHAT NOT TO EAT

Processed foods, foods from fast food outlets, crisps, chips, cakes, biscuits, chocolate, ice-cream, bread, alcohol, sugar in all its forms: including honey, starchy vegetables, potato (skins excepted), yams, beetroot, parsnip, peas

Fruits — watermelon, mangoes and most other fruit

Low-fat foods — like low-fat yoghurt

Oils — vegetable and seed oils (safflower, canola, rapeseed, sunflower)

Drinks — all fruit juices, fizzy drinks and diet fizzy drinks

Sauces — tomato ketchup, brown, BBQ, chilli (contain huge amounts of sugar)

Figure 16.2. What to eat, and what not to eat.

THE SUGAR SIRENS

Have a peek in your larder. Do you see biscuits, crisps, fruit juices, cereals and other packaged foods? You are stocked up on poisons, not food; food does not come in a packet. And now you understand the consequences for you and your loved ones. Have you ever intended to eat 'just one biscuit', but instead eaten the whole packet? We certainly have, and it's neither our fault nor yours. Corporate 'Big Food' designs it that way.

In Homer's *Odyssey*, Odysseus, bravest of heroes, was chained to his ship's mast so he could resist the call of the sirens. Like the sirens, these seductive foods will sit in your larder inviting you to eat them. But unlike Odysseus you can't chain yourself to the mast.

You, like him, are captivated by the lure of the sirens – in this case the sugar sirens – but you must resist. Look at the biscuits, the crisps and cereals. Know that they are making you ill, and making it impossible to lose weight. And do not even consider giving them away. Do the right thing. Garbage belongs in the garbage bin.

****THROW THE PROCESSED FOOD OUT ****

Now is the time to start. You now understand the road that got you here, and you have seen the road map to get you out. You are armed with knowledge about the foods that you are going to eat, how much of each one to eat and what you are not going to eat.

CONGRATULATIONS ☺

You are now ready to draw up your action plan, identify people to follow it with you, tell your family and friends, and set your date for day 1, week 1. Take your 'before' photos (and remember to take the 'after' ones in 12 weeks' time).

From all of us at Whisperer HQ, from the bottom of our hearts, we wish you good luck. You will look and feel the 'new you' very soon. Remember to let us know how you do.

CHAPTER WHISPERINGS

- We use a low-carb, high-fat diet as a springboard into fat adaptation.
- The macronutrient composition that we recommend is C5:F70:P25.

- Keto flu causes a variety of symptoms including headaches, foggy brain and lethargy.
- Keto flu last typically for up to a week, although it can last longer. But it will pass.
- Measures to prevent keto flu include rest, sleep, light stretching exercise and a slow introduction of the keto diet.
- Adequate hydration is important on a low-carb, high-fat diet.
- You may drink water, black tea, green or unsweetened herbal tea (no milk) and black coffee.
- Restrictive diets are not suitable for everyone, and you should check with your doctor if you have a long-term illness or take medications.
- A high-quality low-carb, high-fat diet has real, not processed food.

17

THE 12-WEEK RESET PLAN: WEEKS 1–4

Gentlemen, start your engines!

Tony Hulman, Indy 500

You have now learned the ground rules. You have gained all the knowledge required to apply the *whisperer-loss plan* to yourself, your family and friends. You now understand what makes you put on weight, how to change your body to a fat-burning engine and how to lose weight permanently.

	MON	TUE	WED	THU	FRI	SAT	SUN
Meals	3	3	3				
EatSpan hrs	16	14	12				
FastSpan hrs	8	10	12				
Carbs g	51	28	50				
Fats g	136	150	132				
Protein g	90	120	75				
Weight lb/kg	142	141	141				

Figure 17.1. Weight loss journal; daily entries for week 1. Some people find this a great motivator. It is also helpful to total your EatSpan and FastSpan for comparisons, week to week.

You have finished all the preparation: set your goals, calculated your macronutrients, done your measurements and started your weight loss journal. You know your basal metabolic rate and the amount of each macronutrient by weight per day for your low-carb, high-fat diet. You have documented all your baseline parameters (Figure 15.2). Now is the time to start your weight loss journey and get your fat-burning engine going.

On Sunday every week, sit down and plan your week ahead. The plans are quite didactic but are simple to follow. Make sure you track your food daily, and fill in your weight loss journal (Figure 17.1).

WEEK 1

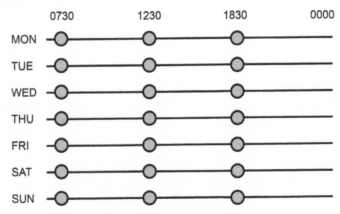

Figure 17.2. EatSpan and FastSpan for *Whisperer-loss* week 1. Total meals per week = 21.

Food

- Carbs: fat: protein in the ratio C5:F70:P25. Keep carbs at or below your target level, under 50 grams per day and sometimes less.
- An overview of the plans is available at the end of Chapter 20 (Figures 20.5, 20.6 and 20.7).
- Eat the amount of food in grams as calculated in your macronutrient composition and do not eat more than that (see Chapter 16 'Understanding Keto Diet Numbers').
- No refined or super-refined carbs. For help on what to eat and not to eat refer to Figure 16.2).
- No snacking before or after meals, or between last meal and breakfast.

- Minimum three litres of fluid per day in the form of unsweetened black coffee, black, green or unsweetened herbal tea or water.
- In the first few weeks, if you find carbohydrate withdrawal tough, an occasional whole fruit may be eaten, such as an apple. We call this your 'rescue apple'. Give yourself five apples for emergencies in the first week.
- Stop drinking alcohol.
- Total meal number = 21.

EatSpan and FastSpan
- Three meals per day, taken at any time.
- Please note: if you normally skip breakfast, don't suddenly start eating it now; stick to a two-meal-a-day regime, with no snacking.

When you have completed week 1:
- You are getting to grips with the macronutrients and finding the whole process of mealtimes a little easier.
- Some people have dramatic weight loss after one week, which can vary from losing 1 to 10 pounds (0.5 to 4.5 kg).
- Don't be disappointed if your partner loses more weight than you do. Weight loss is related to percentage of your body mass and the larger you are, the more likely that you will trump the weight loss stakes in term of kilograms lost; but in terms of percentages, the results may be quite even.
- Ketosis starts when you have used up all your carb stores, which can take up to three days. The point at which you become ketotic depends on the amount of carbs you had in storage when you started, your level of activity, the amount that you move, and how low in carbs your diet is. But you should certainly be ketotic by the end of week 1.
- Once you become ketotic, you may develop keto flu (Figure 16.1).
- You and others may smell ketones on your breath.
- Depending on the strength of your carb addiction, you may have food cravings; use your strategies to deal with this.

WEEK 2

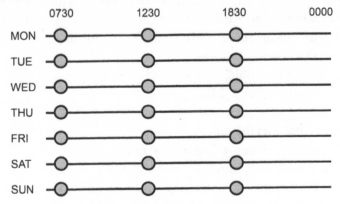

Figure 17.3. EatSpan and FastSpan for *Whisperer-loss* week 2. Total meals per week = 21.

Food
- Unchanged.
- Three rescue apples permitted for the week.
- Total meal number = 21.

EatSpan and FastSpan
- Three meals per day taken at any time.

When you have completed week 2:
- It is important to ensure that you stick to the maximum daily macronutrients by weight.
- Adjust the meal plan to suit your tastes.
- You will now have lost weight, but this is still variable and can zigzag at first and a lot of initial weight loss is water. So be patient.
- You may still have keto flu, but it should be lessening, at least have plateaued. You may still be moody, so ask others for support and help.
- You and other people may smell ketones on your breath.
- If you are not ketotic, look at your carb intake and ensure that you are keeping it low.
- You may be very thirsty; listen to your body and keep hydrated.
- You may have intense cravings; sugar addiction is a hard one to

break. Resist the sugars sirens and use your pre-planned tactics to deal with this.

- The first two weeks are probably the hardest time. Very well done and keep at it!

WEEK 3

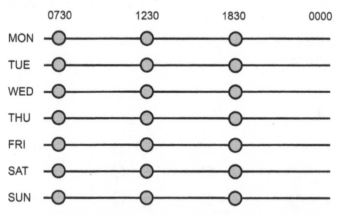

Figure 17.4. EatSpan and FastSpan for *Whisperer-loss* week 3. Total meals per week = 21.

Food
- Unchanged.
- 1 rescue apple permitted for the week.
- Total meal number = 21.

EatSpan and FastSpan
- Three meals per day.

When you have completed week 3:
- You may feel like experimenting a little with your foods, and you now have a good feel for foods that work with your calculated macronutrient composition and those that don't.
- You will now start to see a weight loss of 1 to 2 pounds (0.5 to 1 kg), depending on your size. You also feel that your body is changing.
- Your waist and waist–hip ratio have started to reduce. These are the most important metrics and are more indicative of metabolic health than your weight.

- The keto flu has resolved.
- You're accustomed to the ketones on your breath.
- You may be very thirsty; keeping hydrated is important.
- Carb cravings may intermittently rear their ugly head – be strong, you've got this far now, you can carry on.
- If you are not ketotic, it is time to re-valuate. The four reasons are **a)** You are eating more than 25–50 g of carbs per day, **b)** protein is too high, **c)** fats are too low or **d)** you're eating too much!
- If you have not lost weight, the three possibilities are stress, poor sleep and snacking.

WEEK 4

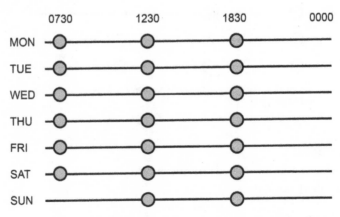

Figure 17.5. EatSpan and FastSpan for *Whisperer-loss* week 4. Total meals per week = 20.

Food
- Unchanged.
- Zero rescue apples this week!
- Total meal number = 20.

EatSpan and FastSpan
- This week you will skip breakfast on Sunday; it will be your first fast of 16 hours.
- Three meals per day.

When you have completed week 4:

- You are enjoying your food more and you can now experiment with different foods.
- You will start to see a weight loss of 1 to 2 pounds (0.5 to 1 kg) this week.
- You now feel that your body is changing. Your waist measurement has reduced.
- Keto flu has resolved.
- You're accustomed to the ketones on your breath.
- Carb cravings and the sugar sirens continue to rear their ugly heads – be strong, you've got to here, you can carry on.
- You may be very thirsty and keeping hydrated is important.
- At the end of week 4, you fasted for 16 hours, your first real fast. This will torch your fat stores and is the start of significant weight loss. Very well done. 😊

CHAPTER WHISPERINGS

- Ensure all preparations are completed before starting your 12-week plan.
- Eat a low-carb 5 per cent, high-fat 70 per cent, moderate-protein 25 per cent diet.
- Calculate your macronutrient composition in grams and do not exceed these amounts.
- Eat three meals per day (unless you habitually eat fewer meals, in which case stay on that regime).
- The shorter your EatSpan and the longer your FastSpan, the greater the weight loss.
- No snacking.
- Eat high-quality, real food, organic if possible.
- Avoid processed foods.
- Eat mindfully.
- Identify your cravings and use pre-planned strategies to deal with them.
- If motivation wanes, revisit your goals.
- Measure your metrics regularly.

18

THE 12-WEEK RESET PLAN: FASTING FITNESS

> In the afternoon the digestion of the meal deprives me of the incomparable lightness which characterises the fast days.
>
> Adalbert de Vogüé

We outlined the hormonal changes associated with *fasting* and *calorie restriction* in Chapter 10, showing the great differences between them. Fasting is a natural state for the body; we are designed to fast and use our fat energy stores in times of need. In contrast, calorie restriction is a stress situation, where the body uses every trick in the book to avoid using its fat stores and preserve your weight.[1]

In your *12-week reset plan*, we have chosen to introduce fasting slowly now that you are fat adapted. Your first four weeks of low carbs will have reignited your fat fuelling engine and now allow you to introduce fasting to your weight loss regime, in a gentle way. We will gradually build up the periods of fasting, which makes it easier, both mentally and physically. When you fast, you will be fuelling entirely on your fat stores. This means fat loss, and the longer you fast, the greater the weight loss. It's like anything; the more you do it, the easier it gets. You will be fasting fit when you have completed your *12-week reset plan!*

HOW TO GET FASTING FIT

1. Think positively about fasting. You will learn to relax and do less.
2. Like running, it is an effort initially, both physically and mentally, but you have all the tools to achieve successful fasting. Don't give up.
3. Everyone can be *fasting fit*. Our ancestors had periods of food scarcity and we descended from those very same people, inheriting their genes.
4. Fasting is a natural part of your constitution, your body and mind have just never been trained.
5. The amount in each meal remains the same and you should keep your portion sizes as before (see Chapter 16).
6. Avoid overeating after a fast. Eat a normal-sized meal, slowly, mindfully, without distractions (TV), stopping when you're 80 per cent full (remember *Hara Hachi Bu*).
7. It is very important to stay hydrated. As food contains 20 per cent of your fluid intake, you will need to increase this to compensate for the loss of water when you are eating less food. Men need 6 pints per day (3.3 litres), and women 4 pints (2.3 litres) per day. One technique for increasing hydration is to drink a pint of water on waking. Store tap water in a glass screw-top or clip-top bottle in the fridge for a refreshing start to the day.
8. If you don't exercise, do not start now (see Chapter 12).
9. If you're already exercising, continue unchanged. At the beginning, stretching, walking or yoga on fasting days may help. As you become increasingly fat adapted, you may get some benefit from training in the fasted state; this speeds up your fat adaptation, and growth hormone is elevated during fasting, which aids recovery.[2] For ultra-runners this will become part of your endurance fat adaptation.
10. Prepare for your fasting day by avoiding all alcohol the night before. If you try to fast on the day after a big night out, you will struggle and make it impossibly difficult for yourself.
11. If you are the only one in your house following a fasting regime, it is difficult to see others eating. Have a strategy for this; persuade

your partner to fast with you, or plan what to do when others are eating. At work, if everyone eats at their desk and you are skipping lunch, consider going out for a walk instead.

12. You can change your fasting days within each week to suit your lifestyle. It will be easier on you if you fast on a more gentle, quiet day.

13. No need to lose your friends; after week 8 use your treat meals to fit in with your life. The timing of your treat meals can be altered to suit social events and other commitments. But ensure that you do not eat super-refined carbs. Very few people notice if you skip the pudding. You can have the cheese, but quietly skip the crackers or bread.

14. Occasionally, you will give up on your fast. Your body says no, your mind says no, or your life intervenes. Listen to your body, reduce the fasting duration and regroup. No worries. Now is not the time to freak out and eat rubbish food. Ask for help from your support group. Dust yourself down, eat one of your favourite keto meals and carry on. Repeat the week where you missed the fast. Do not give up, everyone has hiccups, including everyone at Whisperer HQ.

15. Hunger, brain fog and irritability will gradually decrease as your fat adaptation improves. Your fasting fitness improves as you do more prolonged fasts.

16. Be patient. Fat adaptation happens quickly at first but continues to improve for up to 18 months (Figure 18.1). The more fasting you do, the easier it gets.

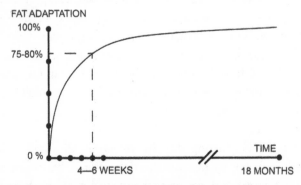

Figure 18.1. The timescale of fat adaptation. Beginning with your ketogenic springboard, then intermittent fasting. 75% of fat adaptation occurs very quickly, with the last 20—25% taking 12—18 months.

17. Once you are fully fat adapted, it is very easy to do long fasts and they become strangely enjoyable. We genuinely look forward to our longer fasts.

18. Once you have done a long fast, it is a good tactic to have a strategy for breaking it. Plan your meal carefully; remember you are still eating a keto diet. Your meal should be a normal sized one.

19. Remember it takes 20 minutes for your satiety hormones to tell your brain that you have eaten enough; you might like to have a small first course and then wait for 20 minutes before eating your main course.

20. Once you have finished the 12-week plan, you can incorporate fasting into your life to improve your metabolism and give you permanent weight control. Fasting is part of the *whisperer-stable plan*; it will control your weight and has significant health benefits and anti-ageing effects. And fasting is part of the *whisperer-recover plan* should you go AWOL.

Please note

1. Fasting is not for everyone; pregnant women and those breast-feeding should avoid it. Do not involve your children or teenagers in fasting regimes; they need nutrition to grow, and you now know very well the foods they need.

2. There are many variables in fasting practices and there is little scientific agreement on the optimal method to achieve weight loss, disease reversal and healthy ageing.[3,4] At present, there are no hard and fast rules about fasting, although this will come in distant future.[5] Our guidance uses the best available current scientific knowledge, combined with our experience in helping others.[6] We suggest that you follow the whisperer plan for fasting as outlined; once you have achieved your targets, you can then perhaps experiment with other fasting techniques.

CHAPTER WHISPERINGS

- Fasting is very different to calorie restriction.
- Fasting is a natural human state.
- Everyone can learn to fast.
- Fat adaptation allows fasting without multiple physical problems.
- Fasting requires mental and physical training.
- Fasting fitness improves with time.
- Don't change your exercise regime when you introduce fasting.
- Do not change the amount eaten at remaining meals. Three meals do not become one!
- Ensure that you are well hydrated and drink enough when fasting.
- Do not drink alcohol before a fasting day.
- Your fasting fitness improves for up to 12–18 months.
- Fasting is good for weight loss, disease reversal and better ageing.

19

THE 12-WEEK RESET PLAN: WEEKS 5–8

Nature does not hurry, yet everything is accomplished
Lao Tzu, circa 500 BC

WEEK 5

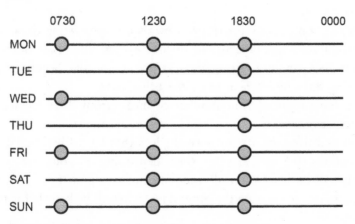

Figure 19.1. EatSpan and FastSpan for *Whisperer-loss* week 5.
Total meals per week = 18

Food

- Carbs: fat: protein unchanged at C5:F70:P25. Keep those carbs under your allowance, usually between 25 and 50 grams.
- An overview of the plans is available at the end of Chapter 20 (Figures 20.5, 20.6 and 20.7).
- Do not just move the food from your breakfast to the residual meals on your fasting days, keep portions the same size as before, do not replace the lost meal and do not put three meals into two.

- No refined or super-refined carbs.
- No snacking, before or after meals, or between last meal and breakfast.
- Three litres of fluid per day in the form of black coffee, tea or water.
- Refrain from drinking alcohol.
- Total meal number = 18.

EatSpan and FastSpan
- Three meals per day for most days.
- You will skip breakfast on three mornings.
- Your FastSpan will increase for three days, and your hormones can now burn through fat.
- Your EatSpan will decrease for these three days.

When you have completed week 5:
- You are now seeing amazing progress; your EatSpan is down and FastSpan is up.
- Do not compensate for skipped meals on non-fasting days, keep portion sizes unchanged and do not exceed your macronutrient allowance on non-fasting days. Don't undo the benefit of the fasting days by overeating on the other days.
- You have reduced your number of meals from three to two for three days.
- You will now see a steady weight loss that varies between 1 and 2 pounds (0.5 to 1 kg) per week, depending on your size.
- You will be ketotic on all your fasting days and, providing that you do not overeat on the other days, you will be ketotic for those days too.
- Your carb addiction is lessening. Carb cravings may still rear their ugly head but be strong.
- You will find that hunger is not one of the major sensations during your fasts.
- Carry on with your weight loss journal.
- Now you are making tangible progress. Well done.

WEEK 6

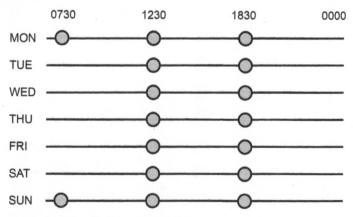

Figure 19.2. EatSpan and FastSpan for *Whisperer-loss* week 6.
Total meals per week = 16.

Food

- Unchanged.
- Total meal number = 16.

EatSpan and FastSpan

- Three meals per day for two days.
- You will skip breakfast on five days.
- Your FastSpan increases on five days.
- Your EatSpan decreases on these five days.

When you have completed week 6:

- You have reduced your weekly total number of meals from an initial 21 meals a week to 16 meals per week, a big achievement.
- You EatSpan continues to reduce and your FastSpan to increase.
- Carry on with your previous macronutrient composition.
- Do not eat the equivalent of three meals in a two-meal day; keep your portion sizes as they were.
- Weigh yourself every day on waking, after emptying your bladder but before you drink anything, naked or in the same clothes every time.
- Complete your weight loss journal including your weight and watch your life change, see how much nearer you are to your goals compared to when you started!
- You are making great progress. Well done.

WEEK 7

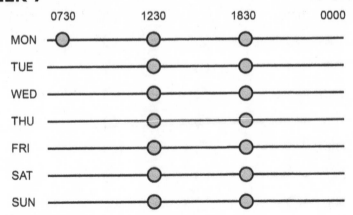

Figure 19.3. EatSpan and FastSpan for *Whisperer-loss* week 7.
Total meals per week = 15.

Food
- Unchanged.
- Total meal number = 15.

EatSpan and FastSpan
- Three meals per day for one day.
- You will skip breakfast on six days.
- Your FastSpan increases on these six days.
- Your EatSpan decreases on these six days.

When you have completed week 7:
- Don't forget to keep your daily EatSpan and FastSpan hours and tot them up at the end of the week.
- You have stopped eating breakfast. You are probably not missing it at all now. Great progress.
- Make sure that you do not have an extra helping at lunch to compensate for skipping breakfast. Do not replace breakfast with bigger meals later that day.
- Your weight loss is continuing.
- You are not hungry; you may have some keto symptoms, but these are only intermittent.
- The sugar sirens still call to you. Try imagining how bad sugar is for you and really start to dislike what sugar has put you through.
- Seven weeks on, your waist is smaller; look back at your journal

and see the difference. Carry on: your waist will continue to shrink as your weight loss progresses. Your waist-to-hip ratio and ABSI will also have reduced and may now be in the normal range, or at least heading there.

- Great work! Keep going – you can do it.

WEEK 8

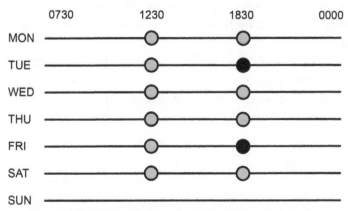

Figure 20.1. EatSpan and FastSpan for *Whisperer-loss* week 9. Total meals per week = 12 (Two treat meals).

Food
- Unchanged.
- Total meal number = 13.

EatSpan and FastSpan
- Two meals a day on all except one day.
- On one day you will not only skip breakfast, but lunch too.
- That means you will do your first 24-hour fast. This is a big and significant day.
- Try your best to reduce your EatSpan, thereby increasing your FastSpan as well. This means eating lunch later and supper earlier. Even 30–60 minutes will make a difference, as your weekly totals will show.

When you have completed week 8:

- You have finished the second four-week block; only one left to go. Very well done.
- You have now kicked the breakfast habit. A big milestone. Paul and I have not eaten breakfast for about three years. Humans don't need three meals a day. Time to celebrate; you will never look back.
- Have a look at your figures, especially EatSpan and FastSpan. EatSpan and total meals are down and FastSpan is up. Well done you!
- Your weight loss journal now has a two-month story, and it should fill you with pride.
- Keep the faith – you have your first treat meal next week.
- Onwards and upwards! Carry on, you're doing well. 😊

20

THE 12-WEEK RESET PLAN: WEEKS 9–12

There are no shortcuts to any place worth going.
Helen Keller, 1880–1968

WEEK 9

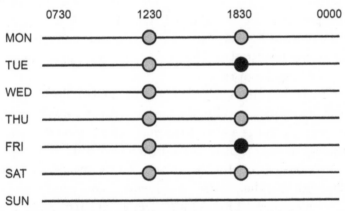

Figure 20.1. EatSpan and FastSpan for *Whisperer-loss* week 9. Total meals per week = 12 (Two treat meals).

Food

- Carbs: fat: protein unchanged at C5:F70:P25 for all but two treat meals.
- An overview of the plans is available at the end of this chapter.
- Macronutrients amounts reduced according to your (new) weight-adjusted BMR.
- Three litres of fluid per day in the form of black coffee, tea or water.

- Two treat meals, with alcohol should you so desire.
- You should really enjoy your treat meals!
- Total meal number = 12.

EatSpan and FastSpan
- Two meals each day, leading up to a 42-hour fast.
- FastSpan is the longest yet, with a single fast for 42 hours, from Saturday evening meal until Monday lunchtime. Wow! Mitochondria will be renewing as autophagy is turned on.
- Your EatSpan is decreasing and FastSpan increasing.

When you have completed week 9:
- It is one of the greatest moments in your life when you realise that you can fast without hunger or symptoms, and finally you know your metabolic health is returning.
- You can choose whichever days you like for your long fast, it just needs to be a continuous 42 hours.
- You have two treat meals to look forward to, which can be lunch or supper, and you are allowed refined carbohydrates in these meals. You can for the treat meal ignore your carb allowance in your macronutrient plan. This means that you can eat foods such as potato, pasta and rice.
- Your treat meal does not include any super-refined carbs. No sweets, no muffins, no chocolate, no pastries; they will play havoc with your hormones and undo so much of the good that you have done. You now recognise this stuff for what it is. Garbage!
- You may have alcohol with your meal. Champagne, or a shot of vodka with sparkling water, or red wine. Many people get caught out, so please be VERY, VERY careful, and remember you are lighter now and you have not had a drink for eight weeks.
- After your treat meal you will not be ketotic for a while, perhaps a day. It's quite good for your body to have a change. Ketosis will soon return as you resume your normal food and fasting regime.
- The sugar sirens may reappear; remember how you managed them before. Have some cheese, or berries and lovely full-fat cream!

WEEK 10

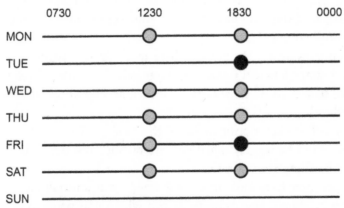

Figure 20.2. EatSpan and FastSpan for *Whisperer-loss* week 10. Total meals per week = 11 (Two treat meals).

Food
- Carbs: fat: protein C5:F70:P25 for all but two treat meals.
- Three litres of fluid per day in the form of black coffee, tea or water.
- Two treat meals.
- Total meal number = 11.

EatSpan and FastSpan
- Two meals per day, on five days.
- One fast for 24 hours from Monday evening to your treat meal on Tuesday evening.
- At the end of this week, you have your second 42-hour fast.

When you have completed week 10:
- Your first 42-hour-plus fast was last week. You have done two further fasts this week; one 24-hour and one 42-hour fast. Mentally and physically, fasting is no big deal by now.
- Breakfast is a distant memory, and you never miss it.
- Your default routine is now two meals per day.
- Our biological clocks respond better to food earlier in the day. We made the plans to best fit in with people who work, but it is perfectly OK to change the timings to suit you. If you would rather have breakfast and lunch, no problem. Or have the treat

meals at lunchtime instead of the evening – great. And try to keep a rhythm, so your body knows what to expect. Chopping and changing is not ideal, as body clocks need to adapt too!

- Make sure that you have finished your supper three to four hours before bedtime.
- Do not overeat – do not eat three meals in one sitting.
- Your shape has really changed, your belly is smaller, you have lost a lot of weight, your clothes are looser, and you now fit your 'thin clothes'!
- You will be ketotic for much of the time.
- You won't be hungry when you are fasting, and the carb cravings will be disappearing now.
- Spend some time looking at your weight loss journal; look at your journey, where you came from and where you want to go. Look at the reduction in EatSpan, in number of meals, your waist measurement, your waist–hip ratio and ABSI, and give yourself a pat on the back.
- Enjoy your treat meals, but don't overdo it, and no super-refined carbs.
- You are nearly there; keep going!

WEEK 11

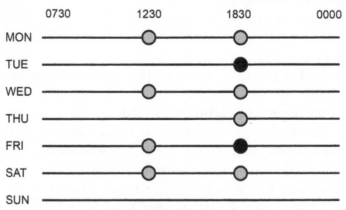

Figure 20.3. EatSpan and FastSpan for *Whisperer-loss* week 11. Total meals per week = 10 (Two treat meals).

Food

- Carbs: fat: protein C5:F70:P25 for all but two treat meals.
- Three litres of fluid per day in the form of black coffee, tea or water.
- Two treat meals.
- Total meal number = 10.

EatSpan and FastSpan

- Two meals a day for four days.
- Two 24-hour fasts during the week.
- One 48-hour fast at the end of the week.

When you have completed week 11:

- On four days you will be eating only two meals each day, at lunch and in the evening, with breakfast now completely omitted from your diet. This week you will miss three lunches too.
- Enjoy your treat meals.
- You may be able to adjust the fasting regime to sync with your body clock. Eating earlier in the day means a healthier hormonal response than eating the same meal later; so if your lifestyle allows, on the days with one meal, instead of skipping lunch and eating supper, you could eat lunch and skip supper.
- As a rule, and this is applicable for the rest of your life too, if you come to any mealtime and don't feel hungry, don't eat. Only foolish rules state we eat when we don't need or want to. But don't turn this skipped meal into a snack later.
- Your weight is falling by 1–2 pounds (0.5 to 1 kg) per week. You will notice now that your shape has changed considerably.
- Keep your weight loss journal entries going; your weight, waist–hip ratio, ABSI, EatSpan, FastSpan and number of meals. It will really help you to see what you have achieved and to help others. Becoming a whisperer is about getting the message out there and helping others. It's great karma for you too.
- One week to go of this journey; you have nearly done it! Feel proud.

WEEK 12

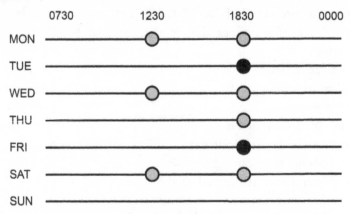

Figure 20.4. EatSpan and FastSpan for *Whisperer-loss* week 12. Total meals per week = 9 (Two treat meals).

Food

- Carbs: fat: protein C5:F70:P25 for all but two treat meals.
- Three litres of fluid per day in the form of black coffee, tea or water.
- Two treat meals.
- On three days this week you will be eating only two meals each day. You will miss four lunches too, meaning OMOD, or *one meal once daily.*
- Total meal number = 9.

EatSpan and FastSpan

- Two meals per day for three days.
- Two 24-hour fasts.
- At the end of this week, you have a 48-hour fast until Monday.

When you have completed week 12:

- This is where we hand over and you take the controls. Your future journey advice is in the next chapter.
- You now utilise all the skills you've learned to create your own path going forwards, enjoying your fasting days as much as your food days. This balance will stay with you for life, completely changing your relationship with food and giving you the power to control your weight and gain a fantastic hormonal balance, as well as a sense of physical and mental wellbeing.

- If you *still have more weight to lose*, revisit your weight loss journal, start a new project, establish your new goals, and *repeat the last four-week block, weeks 9–12*. You can continue to repeat this *four*-week block until you are where you want to be.
- You have completed your whisperer plan, lost weight, dropped a dress size (or three), reduced your abdominal girth and regained wellness.
- All those food cravings are now under control; the sugar sirens will always be there, but you are now deaf to their calls.
- Please do let us know how you've done.
- Remember, revisit the quiz – and don't forget your 'after' photos!
- Well done and congratulations. You are very welcome to the Whisperer family, new whisperer 😄

> No one saves us but ourselves.
> No one can and no one may.
> We ourselves must walk the path.
> Buddha Gautama, fifth century BC

The whisperer has shown you the way, we have not saved you; you saved yourself and you yourself walked the path.

Once you have completed the plan, why not share with your family and friends? Worldwide, people's health is in a parlous state, and health services are buckling. Help others to help themselves and improve your karma. You are now a diet whisperer, and you can contribute to solving this worldwide problem.

WHISPERER-LOSS PLAN SUMMARY

	Week 1	Week 2	Week 3	Week 4
Macro C5:F70:P25	Yes	Yes	Yes	Yes
Refined carbs	No	No	No	No
Super-refined carbs	No	No	No	No
Snacks	No	No	No	No
Daily 2—3 litres fluids	Yes	Yes	Yes	Yes
Rescue apple	5	3	1	0
Alcohol	No	No	No	No
Breakfasts	7	7	7	6
Lunches	7	7	7	7
Evening meals	7	7	7	7
Meals per week	21	21	21	20
Treat meals per week	0	0	0	0

Figure 20.5. Weeks 1—4 of the whisperer-loss plan.

WHISPERER-LOSS PLAN SUMMARY

	Week 5	Week 6	Week 7	Week 8
Macro C5:F70:P25	Yes	Yes	Yes	Yes
Refined carbs	No	No	No	No
Super-refined carbs	No	No	No	No
Snacks	No	No	No	No
Daily 2—3 litres fluids	Yes	Yes	Yes	Yes
Rescue apple	No	No	No	No
Alcohol	No	No	No	No
Breakfasts	4	2	1	0
Lunches	7	7	7	6
Evening meals	7	7	7	7
Meals per week	18	16	15	13
Treat meals per week	0	0	0	0

Figure 20.6. Weeks 5—8 of the whisperer-loss plan.

WHISPERER-LOSS PLAN SUMMARY

	Week 9	Week 10	Week 11	Week 12
Macro C5:F70:P25	Yes	Yes	Yes	Yes
Refined carbs	Treats	Treats	Treats	Treats
Super-refined carbs	No	No	No	No
Snacks	No	No	No	No
Daily 2—3 litres fluids	Yes	Yes	Yes	Yes
Rescue apple	No	No	No	No
Alcohol	Treats	Treats	Treats	Treats
Breakfasts	0	0	0	0
Lunches	6	5	4	3
Evening meals	6	6	6	6
Meals per week	12	11	10	9
Treat meals per week	2	2	2	2

Figure 20.7. Weeks 9—12 of the whisperer-loss plan. In these four weeks, longer 48-hour periods of fasting are achieved. Note that some refined carbohydrates and alcohol are allowed with treat meals.

21

THE 12-WEEK RESET PLAN:
WHAT NEXT?

The future depends on what you do today.

Mahatma Gandhi

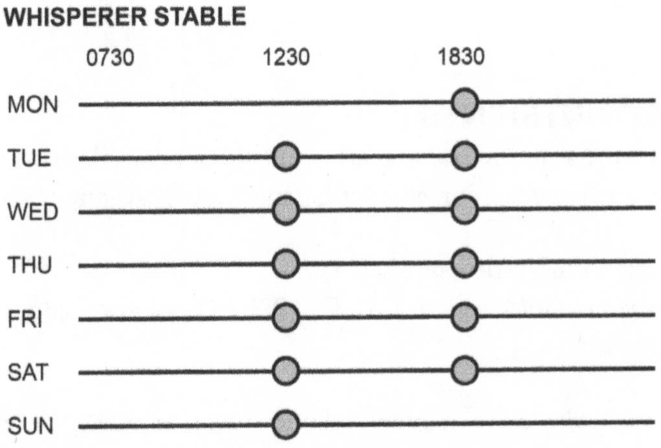

WHISPERER STABLE

Figure 21.1. EatSpan and FastSpan for *Whisperer-stable*. Total meals per week = 12.

SPREAD YOUR WINGS AND FLY FREE AS A BIRD

Now you have your wings, and you're flying solo. You now have the confidence to mix and match your meals and fasts. You know the principles of keeping your EatSpan under 10 hours and your FastSpan over 14 hours. You know the benefits too. 😀

You will be eating two meals a day and helping your body clocks maintain a healthy circadian rhythm. You will have a treat meal when you wish, but in the main eat whole nutritious food, with lots and lots of fibre for your gut bugs. And you will eat mindfully. Fill your plate with fibre, and then add protein and fat.

You have learned to avoid super-refined carbs and processed foods. You may want to switch your fasting from mornings to evenings. This is now all in your hands.

We like to have one 24- to 48-hour fast per week, and one longer fast for 48–72 hours once a month, which we find reinvigorates us.

You may encounter wither of theses circumstances. Firstly, if your weight remains stable, simply continue with your 12 weekly meals. You may increase or decrease the number of weekly meals until you find your equilibrium. This is the *whisperer-stable plan.*

Should you find your weight increases and you need to lose a few pounds quickly, simply repeat weeks 9–12. This we call *whisperer-recover.* If you find yourself in a deeper hole, you may increase the power of your recovery, by repeating weeks 5–8. You will now have the skills to decide.

MACRONUTRIENTS

We suggest that in the stable phase, you should consider two macro-nutrient profiles for your healthy balance nutrition long-term.

For people doing little exercise:
- *Whisperer-stable-regular*: C40:F40:P20. (Carbs are predominantly fibrous greens)

For people who have manual labour intensive work, or exercise frequently:
- *Whisperer-stable-active*: C30:F30:P40. (Carbs are predominantly fibrous greens)

Most people find that somewhere between these two works well for them, and that's fine. Super-refined carbohydrates are not allowed, as they will send you back to where you started. Refined carbohydrate, like potatoes, rice, lentils and beans, can now be a part of the long-term plan, and you can monitor their usage with your weight.

These are of course calorie percentages, so use the same website calculators for your *new* BMR, and your daily macronutrients in grams. If you need any help with those figures, refer back to Chapter 16.

> **IMPORTANT**
>
> All long-term restrictive diets have the potential for nutritional deficiencies. We recommend eating whole, nutritious, varied foods. You can now add legumes, beans, lentils, below ground vegetables and whole grains such as quinoa and buckwheat to what was your keto diet. This will provide you with additional fibre, for your all important gut bugs. Try to eat 30 different plants a week. Avoid snacking, processed foods and sugar. By combining this food with careful timing and respecting your body rhythms, sleep and microbiome, you will achieve long-term balance in your weight and wellness.
>
> Good luck from everyone at Whisperer HQ.

22

THE 12-WEEK RESET PLAN: MEAL PLANS AND RECIPES

He who is not satisfied with a little, is satisfied with nothing.

Epicurus, 341–270 BC

We have tabled a meal plan featuring the recipes here, to help you with your 12-week plan. We do hope that you enjoy the recipes and relax – no special culinary skills are required!

The meal plans are not prescriptive; you can follow the plan to the letter, amend it or plough your own furrow and devise your own plan – you choose. Swap meals to different days, repeat meals that you like or substitute them for your own preferences. An important principle is to keep your carb intake below 5 per cent of your total energy intake; you will know the figure in grams from your macro-nutrient allowance.

Any restrictive diet has its problems, and a low-carb diet is no different; it is very easy not to eat enough fibre as there is virtually no fibre in animal products. Try to save your carb intake for fibre-containing foods such as vegetables, seeds and nuts.

Ideally, all ingredients should be fresh, organic preferably and chemical-free, but don't beat yourself up about this; you can only do what you can do. However, olive oil is an ingredient worth investing in. We really believe that you should use extra virgin, cold-pressed olive oil, ideally organic.

We use very few tinned ingredients, but where they are used, ensure that the tins are free of BPA (a known carcinogen). Also check the list of ingredients, as it is very easy for manufacturers to slip in added sugar, which as we have seen can come in a variety of subtle guises.

There is information in the recipes on the macronutrient composition, with net carbs for a serving of each meal. Having established your daily macronutrient composition, you may need to increase or decrease the number of servings, or alter the serving size, depending on your personal needs. When you reach week 4, you will skip your first meal. On this day, you reduce your daily macronutrient allowance by a third. Similarly, you reduce your macronutrient allowance by two thirds when you skip two meals.

We have not given you recipes for treat meals as, by definition, they must be a treat for you, not us! If you are looking for inspiration, in general you can add refined carbs to your meals. So if your treat meal is a roast dinner, you can now include roast potatoes, stuffing, peas and parsnips. Or add brown bread, hash browns, beans and black pudding to your 'Full English', or perhaps a bolognese with real spaghetti?

To avoid repetition, some of the recipes appear elsewhere: e.g. cauliflower mash has its own recipe and is also used in cottage pie. And we have not insulted you by telling you how to do a Sunday roast, poach an egg or grill a chop!

If you have any queries, we are here to help you. You will find a contact form for Whisperer HQ on our website at www.diet-whisperer.com, and we will be delighted to answer your questions.

	Breakfast	CARBS	Lunch	CARBS	Supper	CARBS	Carb Total
1 MON	Crunchy nut granola	6.5	BLT wrap	1.0	Traditional shakshuka	12	19.5
2 TUE	Yoghurt breakfast bowl	9.4	Courgette Frittata	11.5	Cod chorizo with buttery leeks	4.5	24.9
3 WED	NoatMeal porridge	7.3	Greek omelette	3.0	Bolognese with courgetti	14	24.3
4 THU	Poached eggs, salmon & spinach	4.0	Greek salad	11.0	Creamy garlic prawns with asparagus	4.5	19.5
5 FRI	Frittata egg muffin	1.0	Charcuterie and cheese board	3.5	Chicken tikka, mint yoghurt, Turkish salad	18.8	23.3
6 SAT	Full English	8.0	Kippers, bacon and tomatoes	5.5	Greek marinated chicken & Greek salad	11.0	24.5
7 SUN	Yoghurt breakfast bowl	9.4	Shepherd's pie with buttered leeks	10.5	Garlic mushrooms	5.0	26.9
8 MON	NoatMeal porridge	7.3	Spinach omelette	5.8	Greek salad	11.0	24.3
9 TUE	Crunchy nut granola	6.5	Caprese salad	8.0	Pork chop with haricots vert & roast broccoli	8.5	17.8
10 WED	Yoghurt breakfast bowl	9.4	BLT wrap	1.0	Green shakshuka	13.0	23.4
11 THU	Fritatta egg muffin	1.0	Parma wrap	1.0	Salmon fillet with braised fennel	17.5	19.5
12 FRI	NoatMeal porridge	7.3	Tuna and cabbage salad	12.5	Greek marinated chicken & Greek salad	1.0	20.8
13 SAT	Florentine kippers	2.5	Garlic mushrooms, charcuterie board	8.5	Chicken tikka, mint yoghurt, Turkish salad	9.0	20.0
14 SUN	Full English	8.0	Cottage pie	8.5	Salad niçoise	8.0	24.5

Figure 22.1 Meal plan weeks 1 to 2, with net carbs per meal and daily total net carbs.

	Breakfast	CARBS	Lunch	CARBS	Supper	CARBS	Carb Total
15 MON	Yoghurt breakfast bowl	9.4	BLT wrap	1.0	Cod, chorizo, cauliflower mash, green beans	10.0	20.4
16 TUE	Crunchy nut granola	6.5	Cheese omelette	3.0	Sirloin steak garlic mushrooms	5.0	16.5
17 WED	NoatMeal porridge	7.3	Salad niçoise	8.0	Shepherd's pie with buttered leeks	10.5	27.8
18 THU	Crunchy nut granola	6.5	Creamy garlic prawns with asparagus	4.5	Lamb chops, roasted veg	12.0	23.0
19 FRI	Poached egg with salmon	4.0	Caprese salad	8.0	Mackerel fillet, Greek salad	11.0	23.0
20 SAT	Full English	8.0	Parma wrap	1.0	Bolognese with courgetti	14.0	23.0
21 SUN	Fritatta egg muffin	1.0	Roast beef, haricots verts, roast broccoli	8.5	Caprese salad with avocado	10.0	19.5
22 MON	Fritatta egg muffin	1.0	Spinach omelette	5.8	Bolognese with courgetti	14.0	20.8
23 TUE	NoatMeal porridge	7.3	Greek salad	11.0	Pork sausage (100% pork), celeriac mash	5.0	23.3
24 WED	Crunchy nut granola	6.5	Parma wrap	1.0	Salmon fillet with braised fennel	17.5	25.0
25 THU	Crunchy nut granola	6.5	BLT wrap	1.0	Steak with roasted vegetables	12.0	19.5
26 FRI	Scrambled eggs & mushrooms	2.0	Tuna and cabbage salad	12.5	Cottage pie with haricots verts	8.5	26.5
27 SAT	Kippers, bacon and tomatoes	5.5	Caprese salad	8.0	Chicken tikka, mint yoghurt, Turkish salad	9.0	22.5
28 SUN			Roast lamb with green vegetables	8.5	Garlic mushrooms	5.0	13.5

Figure 22.2 Meal plan weeks 3 to 4, with net carbs per meal and daily total net carbs.

BREAKFAST

NOATMEAL PORRIDGE

1 serving
Net carbs: 7.3 g per serving

Ingredients

- 28 g (1 oz/2 tbsp) chia seeds
- 180 ml (¾ cup) raw, unsweetened full-fat coconut milk
- ½ tsp ground cinnamon

Method

- Mix all the ingredients in a bowl with a spoon and place in the fridge overnight.
- Serve straight from the fridge.

Macronutrients per serving

- Calories: 504; Total Carbs: 18.8 g; Net Carbs: 7.3 g; Fat: 45 g; Protein: 10.9 g; Fibre: 11.5 g

Variations

- Substitute almond milk for coconut milk.
- Add 1 tsp of freshly grated ginger.
- Add seeds from 2 green cardamon pods.
- Top with mixed nuts of your choice.
- Top with raspberries, strawberries or blackberries.
- Top with handful of mixed nuts and berries.

YOGHURT BREAKFAST BOWL

1 serving
Net carbs: 9.4 g per serving

Ingredients

- 100 g (3½ oz) full-fat Greek yoghurt
- 100 g (3½ oz/a handful) raspberries
- 30 g (1 oz/a handful) Brazil nuts

Method

- Put the Greek yoghurt in a bowl.
- Top with the raspberries and Brazil nuts.

Macronutrients per serving

- Calories: 438; Total Carbs: 19.7 g; Net Carbs: 9.4 g;
  Fat: 38.4 g; Protein: 16 g; Fibre: 10.3 g

Variations

- Garnish with a sprinkle of chia seeds or flaxseeds.
- Top with mixed nuts.
- Substitute strawberries or blackberries for raspberries.
- Substitute macadamia nuts for Brazil nuts and add 1.5 g to
  net carbs.

POACHED EGG, SMOKED SALMON AND SPINACH

2 servings
Net carbs: 4 g per serving

Ingredients

- 2 very fresh medium free-range eggs
- White wine vinegar
- 30 g (2 tbsp) butter
- 200 g (7 oz) baby spinach
- 200 g (7 oz) smoked salmon
- Sea salt and black pepper

Method

- Crack the eggs into separate ramekins or dishes.
- Fill a saucepan with water – your pan should be at least 5 cm (2 inches) deep. Add a few drops of vinegar and bring the water to a simmer (not boiling) and stir to create a gentle whirlpool.
- Drop one egg carefully into the centre of the whirlpool. Cook for 3–4 minutes, or until the white has set.
- Gently lift out with a slotted spoon and pop into warm water.
- Repeat with the second egg.
- While the eggs are cooking, melt the butter in a frying pan over a medium heat.
- Add the spinach, season with salt and pepper and cook for 1–2 minutes until the leaves have wilted, stirring occasionally with a wooden spoon.
- Divide the spinach between two plates and top with the slices of smoked salmon.
- Remove the eggs from the water and drain on kitchen paper, then place on top of the smoked salmon.
- Garnish with black pepper.

Macronutrients per serving

- Calories: 255; Total Carbs: 4.5 g; Net Carbs: 2 g; Fat: 14 g; Protein: 20 g; Fibre: 2.5 g

SCRAMBLED EGG WITH BACON AND MUSHROOMS

2 servings
Net carbs: 2 g per serving

Ingredients

- 2 tbsp olive oil
- 125 g (4½ oz) mushrooms, sliced
- 8 cherry tomatoes (keep on the vine)
- 2 rashers unsmoked back bacon
- 4 medium free-range eggs

- 15 g (1 tbsp) butter
- 2 tbsp crème fraîche
- Small handful of chopped chives (optional)
- Sea salt and black pepper

Method

- Heat the olive oil in a frying pan over a medium heat.
- Add the mushrooms and tomatoes, season with salt and pepper and fry for a minute until lightly browned; move to one side of the pan and reduce the heat.
- Add the bacon to the other side of the pan and cook until the bacon is lightly browned on both sides, about 2–3 minutes per side, depending on your preference.
- While these are cooking, cook the scrambled eggs. Crack the eggs into a cold saucepan. Do not season at this point, as this can make the eggs go runny. Add the butter to the pan.
- Place over a medium heat and use a rubber spatula to whisk the eggs while increasing to a high heat. Ensure that you keep scraping the eggs from the side of the pan and moving them around, rather like cooking a risotto.
- Remove from the heat and continue to stir with the spatula, then return to the heat, stir. Take them on and off the heat, stirring all the time, until you have a smooth consistency or one that you like.
- Remove from the heat and stir in the salt and pepper, then the chopped chives, if using, then the crème fraiche.
- Divide the scrambled egg between the two plates and top with the mushrooms and then the bacon.
- Garnish with the vine tomatoes.

Macronutrients per serving

- Calories: 411; Total Carbs: 4 g; Net Carbs: 2 g; Fat: 41 g; Protein: 18 g; Fibre: 4 g

THE FULL ENGLISH

1 serving
Net carbs: 8 g per serving

Ingredients

- 45 ml (3 tbsp) olive oil
- 2 rashers unsmoked back bacon
- 2 sausages (100 per cent pork meat; most sausages have 3–4 per cent carbs and chemicals. Read the label carefully or ask your butcher.)
- 100 g (3½ oz) mushrooms, quartered
- 4 or more cherry tomatoes (on the vine is best)
- 2 medium free-range eggs

Method

- Heat 1 tablespoon of the olive oil in a large frying pan.
- Add the bacon and sausages to the pan and fry, turning occasionally, until cooked.
- Remove from the pan and keep warm in a low oven.
- Add the mushrooms and tomatoes to the frying pan and cook until softened, turning occasionally.
- Heat the remaining 2 tablespoons of olive oil in a small non-stick frying pan over a low heat.
- Crack the eggs into the pan and keep the heat low; if you hear fat spitting, the oil is too hot and you will brown the underside and the sunny side will be raw – I call this egg death.
- Spoon the hot oil over the yolks. For us, when the white is cooked but the yolk is still runny, this is cooked. If you like the yolks solid, keep frying the eggs for a few more seconds and wait until they are firm to the touch.
- Assemble the bacon, sausages, mushrooms, tomatoes and eggs on a warm plate. Forget the garnish – after all, it's a fry-up!

Macronutrients per serving

- Calories: 895; Total Carbs: 10 g; Net Carbs: 8 g; Fat: 72 g; Protein: 59 g; Fibre: 2 g

FRITTATA EGG MUFFINS

1 serving, 2 muffins
Net carbs: 1 g per serving

Ingredients

- 15 ml (1 tbsp) olive oil
- 170 g (6 oz) mushrooms, thinly sliced
- 15 g (1 tbsp) butter, plus extra for greasing
- 200 g (7 oz) spinach
- 6 large free-range eggs
- 100 g (3½ oz) grated Cheddar cheese
- Sea salt and black pepper

Method

- Heat the oil in a frying pan over a medium heat.
- Add the mushrooms and cook until softened, about 10 minutes. Remove from the pan and drain off any liquid. Set aside.
- Melt the butter in a saucepan with a lid over a low heat. Add the spinach, stir to coat in the butter and cover until wilted, about 2 minutes. Drain off any liquid and set aside.
- Preheat the oven to 180°C/350°F/Gas mark 4 and grease a muffin tin with butter.
- Beat the eggs in a large bowl and season with salt and pepper.
- Add the cheese, mushrooms and spinach (make sure that you have drained away any excess liquid first).
- Ladle the egg mixture into the greased muffin cups to three-quarters full (this makes 12 muffins), then put into the oven and bake for 25 minutes.
- Remove from the oven and leave to cool before removing from the tin.
- Eat when cold – the muffins will keep for a few days. These are ideal for a quick breakfast or lunch.

Macronutrients per serving

- Calories: 254; Total Carbs: 2 g; Net Carbs: 1 g; Fat: 18 g; Protein: 20 g; Fibre: 1 g

CRUNCHY NUTTY GRANOLA

12 servings
Net carbs: 6.5 g per serving

Ingredients

- 150 g (1 cup) walnuts
- 150 g (1 cup) hazelnuts
- 130 g (1 cup) Brazil and macadamia nuts
- 150 g (1 cup) coconut flakes
- 65 g (2 tbsp) sunflower seeds
- 40 g (2 tbsp) flaxseed
- 20 g (2 tbsp) chia seeds
- 1 tsp ground cinnamon
- 1 tsp ground ginger
- 1 free-range egg white
- 1 tsp vanilla extract
- 80 ml (⅓ cup) coconut oil, gently melted (not hot)

Method

- Preheat the oven to 150°C/300°F/Gas mark 2 and line a shallow baking tray with baking paper.
- Chop the nuts coarsely in food processor or chop roughly by hand.
- Mix the nuts, coconut flakes, seeds and ground spices in a bowl.
- In a separate large bowl, lightly whisk the egg white until foamy.
- Add the vanilla extract and melted coconut oil to the egg white and stir to combine.
- Tip all the dry ingredients into the wet ingredients and stir until everything is combined. You may need to add a little water to ensure that everything is coated.
- Tip the granola mix onto the lined baking tray and spread out and flatten into an even layer. To ensure all the granola is cooked at the same time, arrange with a space in the centre of the tray, otherwise the granola in the middle of the tray will cook last and the rest will be burned.

- Bake for 25–30 minutes until golden brown. Don't overcook, as the nuts will be unpleasant if burned.
- Remove from the oven and allow to cool before breaking up into small pieces. Store in an airtight glass jar.
- Serve with Greek yoghurt or unsweetened almond milk.

Macronutrients per serving

- Calories: 350; Total Carbs: 10.5 g; Net Carbs: 6.5 g; Fat: 32 g; Protein: 6 g; Fibre: 4 g

Variations

- If you don't like your granola crunchy, omit the egg white steps.
- You can use a variety of nuts, but check the carb count if you substitute nuts containing higher carbs, such as cashew nuts.
- Use any spice mix you like.

GRILLED KIPPERS WITH BACON AND TOMATOES

2 servings
Net carbs: 5.5 g per serving

Ingredients

- 2 whole kippers
- 30 g (2 tbsp) butter
- 4 rashers unsmoked back bacon
- 2 medium tomatoes, sliced in half horizontally
- Glug of olive oil
- Black pepper

Method

- Heat the grill to high and line your grill pan with foil (this will make cleaning a lot easier).
- Place the kippers on the grill rack with the skin side down.
- Season with black pepper and dot with the butter, then place 2 rashers of bacon over each kipper.

- Add the halved tomatoes, drizzle with a glug of olive oil and season with salt and pepper.
- Place under grill for 3 minutes, then turn the bacon over and grill for a further 3 minutes.

Macronutrients per serving

- Calories: 426; Total Carbs: 5.5 g; Net Carbs: 5.5 g; Fat: 31 g; Protein: 30 g; Fibre: 0 g

Variation: Florentine Kippers

- Prepare the kippers as above, then serve on a bed of wilted baby spinach and top with a poached egg.

Macronutrients per serving

- Calories: 331; Total Carbs: 4.5 g; Net Carbs: 2.5 g; Fat: 24 g; Protein: 24.5 g; Fibre: 2 g

LUNCH

BASIC OMELETTE

1 serving
Net carbs: 0 g per serving

Ingredients

- 2 medium free-range eggs
- 15 g (1 tbsp) butter
- 1 tsp fresh chopped parsley
- Sea salt and black pepper

Method

- You will need a cast-iron skillet with rounded edges, 15 cm (6 inches) in diameter.
- Break the eggs into a bowl and with a fork, break up the yolks into the whites. Do not beat vigorously.
- Season with salt and pepper.
- Place the skillet over a medium heat.
- When the pan is hot, add the butter and swirl round to completely cover the base, then turn up heat and pour in the eggs.
- Tilt the pan to spread the eggs evenly.
- Use a spoon to draw the edges of the omelette to the centre, tipping the pan so that the liquid egg runs into the channels.

- When the egg is almost set but the surface is still a little liquid, slip a spatula under one side and fold over.
- Cook for 1 further minute, then slide the omelette onto a plate, garnish with the chopped parsley and serve.

Macronutrients per serving

- Calories: 250; Total Carbs: 0 g; Net Carbs: 0 g; Fat: 11 g; Protein: 12 g; Fibre: 0 g

Variation: Omelette fines herbes

- Add 2 tablespoons finely chopped fresh parsley and 1 tablespoon finely chopped chives to the stirred eggs and allow to sit for 30 minutes before cooking. Proceed as above.

GREEK OMELETTE

1 serving
Net carbs: 3 g per serving

Ingredients

- 1 medium tomato, diced
- 3 black kalamata olives, pitted and cut into small pieces
- 60 g (2 oz/4 tbsp) feta cheese, crumbled
- ¼ tsp fresh oregano
- 2 medium free-range eggs
- 15 g (1 tbsp) butter
- 1 tsp fresh chopped parsley (optional)
- Sea salt and black pepper

Method

- You will need a cast-iron skillet with rounded edges, 15 cm (6 inches) in diameter.
- Mix the tomato, olives, feta cheese and oregano in a bowl and set aside.
- Break the eggs into a bowl and with a fork, break up the yolks into the whites. Do not beat vigorously.
- Season with salt and pepper.
- Place the skillet over a medium heat.

- When the pan is hot, add the butter and swirl round to completely cover the base, then turn up heat and pour in the eggs.
- Tilt the pan to spread the eggs evenly.
- Use a spoon to draw the edges of the omelette to the centre, tipping the pan so that the liquid egg runs into the channels. Repeat until the egg starts to set.
- When the egg is set but the surface is still runny, remove the pan from the heat.
- Add the tomato mixture to one half of the omelette.
- Slip a spatula under the unfilled half and gently fold over the first filled half.
- Return the pan to the heat and cook for a further minute to warm the filling, or place in a hot oven for 1–2 minutes.
- Slide the omelette onto a plate.
- Garnish with chopped flat parsley, if using and serve.

Macronutrients per serving

- Calories: 377; Total Carbs: 3 g; Net Carbs: 3 g; Fat: 21 g; Protein: 14 g; Fibre: 0 g

Variation: Cheese Omelette

- Make the omelette as above. Add 60 g (3 oz) grated cheese for the filling such as Cheddar, Gruyère, Emmental or Parmesan.

Variation: Mushroom Omelette

- Stir-fry finely chopped ginger, spring onions and red chillies (to taste). Season. When softened, add mushrooms. Drain off any liquid and set aside. Make the omelette and fill as above. Garnish with coriander.

Variation: Spinach Omelette

- Cook 200 g (7 oz) spinach in butter, season and set aside, draining off any liquid. Make the omelette and fill as above with spinach and grated Gruyère or Parmesan.

FRITTATA

3 servings
Net carbs: 11.5 g per serving

Ingredients

- 30 g (2 tbsp) butter
- 1 white onion, finely chopped
- 1 garlic clove, finely chopped
- 3 medium courgettes, coarsely grated
- 8 large free-range eggs
- 60 ml (¼ cup) single cream
- 100 g (3½oz) grated Cheddar cheese
- Sea salt and black pepper

Method

- Add the butter to an ovenproof cast-iron skillet and place over a medium heat.
- Add the onion, garlic and courgettes to the skillet and soften over a medium heat for a few minutes.
- Preheat the oven to 190°C/375°F/Gas mark 5.
- Whisk the eggs with the cream just until smooth – don't whisk too much.
- Stir in half the grated cheese and season with salt and pepper.
- Add the egg mixture to the vegetables in the pan and tilt to spread the egg mixture evenly.
- Cook over a low heat until the edges have set. This will only take a few minutes.
- Top with the remaining cheese, then transfer to the oven for 20–30 minutes. It is cooked when the centre is set.
- Remove from the oven and allow to stand for 5 minutes, then loosen around the edge and cut into wedges.
- Serve with a green salad.
- Frittata can be eaten cold and will keep for up to a week.

Macronutrients per serving

- Calories: 535; Total Carbs: 14.5 g; Net Carbs: 11.5 g; Fat: 36 g; Protein: 4.5 g; Fibre: 3 g

Variations

- Add chopped cooked bacon or any vegetable such as wilted spinach or cooked mushrooms. Avoid tomatoes, as they can make the mixture too watery.

TUNA AND WHITE CABBAGE SALAD

4 servings
Net carbs: 12.5 g per serving

Ingredients

- 2 x 200 g (7 oz) tins tuna in brine
- 1 red onion, finely diced
- 1 tbsp mayonnaise
- Tabasco (optional)
- White cabbage salad (see page 225)
- 2 x hard-boiled eggs, shelled and each cut into six wedges
- 6 cherry tomatoes, quartered
- Small handful of chopped coriander
- Sea salt and black pepper

Method

- Drain the tuna and place in a bowl.
- Add the red onion, mayonnaise and Tabasco, if using, to taste.
- Season with salt and pepper and mix all the ingredients together.
- Arrange the white cabbage salad in a doughnut shape on each serving plate, leaving an empty well in the middle.
- Spoon the tuna mixture inside the well.
- Place the eggs evenly around the outside of the plate.
- Place the cherry tomatoes between the eggs.
- Finish by scattering with the coriander.

Macronutrients per serving

- Calories: 288; Total Carbs: 17 g; Net Carbs: 12.5 g; Fat: 12.5 g; Protein: 29.5 g; Fibre: 5.5 g

BLT WRAP

1 serving
Net carbs: 1 g per serving

Ingredients

- 15 ml (1 tbsp) olive oil
- 2 rashers unsmoked back bacon
- 2 Romaine or iceberg lettuce leaves
- 1 tbsp mayonnaise
- 1 ripe tomato, sliced
- Sea salt and black pepper

Method

- Pour the olive oil into a frying pan and place over a medium heat.
- Add the bacon rashers and fry until crisp on both sides.
- Meanwhile, 'butter' the lettuce leaves with the mayonnaise.
- Place one rasher on top of each lettuce leaf and top with the tomato slices.
- Fold leaf over and eat as a wrap.
- Be prepared for spillage!

Macronutrients per serving

- Calories: 256; Total Carbs: 5 g; Net Carbs: 5 g; Fat: 23 g; Protein: 7 g; Fibre: 0 g

PROSCIUTTO WRAP

2 servings
Net carbs: 1 g per serving

Ingredients

- 1 avocado
- 1 lime, halved
- Green salad leaves
- 6 slices of Parma ham
- 15 ml (1 tbsp) olive oil
- Sea salt and black pepper

Method

- Cut the avocado lengthways onto the large stone, gently twist and the halves will separate. Remove the stone.
- Remove the avocado skin; if your avocadoes are ripe you should be able to manually separate the skin from the flesh. Alternatively, use a spoon to scoop the avocado flesh out of the skin.
- Slice each avocado half widthways into 5–6 thickish slices, then squeeze the lime over the avocado slices and season with salt and pepper.
- Place the salad leaves on serving plate.
- Lay a slice of Parma ham flat on a separate plate.
- Place 1–2 avocado slices on each slice of Parma ham, then roll up the prosciutto and sliced avocado together.
- Place the prosciutto wraps on top of the salad leaves and drizzle with the olive oil.
- Serve alone or with caprese salad (see page 224).

Macronutrients per serving

- Calories: 272; Total Carbs: 6 g; Net Carbs: 1 g; Fat: 23 g; Protein: 13 g; Fibre: 5 g

CHARCUTERIE AND CHEESE BOARD

2 servings
Net carbs: 3.5 g per serving

Ingredients

- 6 slices of Parma ham
- 6 slices of bresaola
- 60 g (2 oz) Comté
- 60 g (2 oz) Reblochon
- 120 g (½ cup/4 oz) chopped walnuts
- 4 celery sticks, cut into batons (optional)
- 90 g (3 oz/½ cup) mixed olives
- Sprig of fresh thyme, to garnish

Method

- Arrange the meats, cheeses and nuts on a large wooden board.
- Add the celery sticks, if using.
- Place the olives in a separate bowl alongside.
- Garnish with the sprig of thyme.

Macronutrients per serving

- Calories: 663; Total Carbs: 4.5 g; Net Carbs: 3.5 g; Fat: 47 g; Protein: 57 g; Fibre: 1 g

SALADS

ONION RAITA

4 servings
Net carbs: 4.8 g per serving

Ingredients

- 2 red onions, very thinly sliced
- 20 cherry tomatoes, quartered
- ¼ tsp garam masala
- ¼ tsp cayenne pepper
- Handful of freshly chopped coriander
- 15 ml (1 tbsp) olive oil
- Sea salt and black pepper

Method

- Put the onions and tomatoes in a bowl.
- Add the spices and salt and pepper to taste and mix together.
- Scatter over the coriander, drizzle with the olive oil and mix again.
- Transfer to a serving dish, cover and place in the fridge for several hours before serving.
- Serve with chicken tikka (see page 235) or Greek marinated chicken (see page 237).

Macronutrients per serving

- Calories: 55; Total Carbs: 6 g; Net Carbs: 4.8 g;
  Fat: 4 g; Protein: 1 g; Fibre: 1.2 g

TURKISH SALAD

6 servings
Net carbs: 6.5 g per serving

Ingredients

- 10 (1.4 kg/3 lb 2 oz) medium tomatoes
- 1 cucumber
- 3 large handfuls of coriander (including stalks)
- Juice of 1 lemon
- 15 ml (1 tbsp) olive oil
- Sea salt and black pepper

Method

- Place the tomatoes, cucumber and coriander on a large chopping board, reserving a small handful of coriander leaves to garnish.
- Use a very sharp large knife to chop all the ingredients until they are a smooth, even consistency, almost like a salsa. This will probably take about 15 minutes.
- Place in a large salad bowl and add the lemon juice and salt and pepper to taste.
- Drizzle with the olive oil and lightly toss.
- Garnish with the reserved coriander leaves.
- Serve with chicken tikka (see page 235).

Macronutrients per serving

- Calories: 61; Total Carbs: 9.5 g; Net Carbs: 6.5 g;
  Fat: 2 g; Protein: 2 g; Fibre: 3 g

SALAD NIÇOISE

4 servings
Net carbs: 8 g per serving

Ingredients

- 100–200 g (3½–7 oz) rocket or mixed salad leaves
- 4 medium ripe tomatoes, quartered
- 175 g (6 oz) green beans
- 3 hard-boiled eggs, peeled and quartered
- 2 x 200 g (7 oz) tins tuna in brine, drained and broken up into small chunks
- 50 g (2 oz) anchovy fillets
- 50 g (2 oz) kalamata black olives, pitted and quartered
- Sea salt and black pepper
- Vinaigrette dressing (see page 250)

Method

- Place the salad leaves in a large serving bowl.
- Add the tomatoes and green beans to the bowl in layers.
- Tuck the egg quarters into and around the salad and then arrange the tuna evenly on top.
- Arrange the anchovies in a criss-cross pattern and scatter the olives on top.
- Season with salt and pepper and drizzle with vinaigrette dressing.

Macronutrients per serving

- Calories: 279; Total Carbs: 11 g; Net Carbs: 8 g; Fat: 24.5 g; Protein: 37 g; Fibre: 3 g

GREEK SALAD

3 servings
Net carbs: 11 g per serving

Ingredients

- 60 ml (¼ cup) Greek olive oil, plus extra for drizzling

- 1 tbsp red wine vinegar
- 50 g (2 oz) kalamata black olives, deseeded and quartered
- 3 juicy ripe red tomatoes, cut into wedges
- 1 cucumber, cut into thick half-moon slices
- 1 green pepper, sliced
- 1 medium red onion, thinly sliced into half rings
- 200 g (7 oz) feta cheese, crumbled
- 1 tsp dried oregano
- Sea salt

Method

- Whisk the olive oil and red wine vinegar together and set aside.
- Mix the olives, tomatoes, cucumber, green pepper and onion together in a large serving bowl.
- Season with salt, then pour over the oil and red wine vinegar and toss everything together.
- Top with the feta cheese and oregano.
- Drizzle a few drops of olive oil over the feta cheese.
- Eat as a light meal, or with Greek marinated chicken (see page 237) or a grilled mackerel fillet.

Macronutrients per serving

- Calories: 374; Total Carbs: 14 g; Net Carbs: 11 g; Fat: 31 g; Protein: 11 g; Fibre: 3 g

CLASSIC CAPRESE SALAD

2 servings
Net carbs: 8 g per serving

Ingredients

- 4 (460 g/1 lb) fresh ripe tomatoes
- 225–250 g (8–9 oz) mozzarella balls (2 large)
- 15 ml (1 tbsp) olive oil
- Fresh torn basil leaves
- Sea salt and black pepper

Method

- Cut each tomato into 5 slices.
- Cut each mozzarella ball into 5 slices.
- Lay the tomatoes on a large serving plate and season with salt and pepper.
- Lay a mozzarella slice on top of each tomato slice and drizzle generously with olive oil.
- Scatter over the torn basil leaves.
- Serve as a light meal or accompaniment.

Macronutrients per serving

- Calories: 408; Total Carbs: 11 g; Net Carbs: 8 g; Fat: 30 g; Protein: 26 g; Fibre: 3 g

Variation

- Prepare as above and add a sliced avocado to the side.

Macronutrients per serving

- Calories: 528; Total Carbs: 18 g; Net Carbs: 10 g; Fat: 41 g; Protein: 27.5 g; Fibre: 8 g

WHITE CABBAGE SALAD

4 servings
Net carbs: 6.5 g per serving

Ingredients

- ½ white cabbage, very thinly sliced
- 1 white onion, thinly sliced and separated into rings
- ½ iceberg lettuce, thinly sliced
- Juice of 1 lemon
- 15 ml (1 tbsp) olive oil
- Sea salt

Method

- Add the cabbage, lettuce and white onion to a bowl.
- Season with salt and add the lemon juice.

- Drizzle with olive oil and toss everything together.
- Cover and place in fridge for 3–4 hours (it can be eaten straight away but this improves flavour and texture).
- The serving size is generous!

Macronutrients per serving

- Calories: 94; Total Carbs: 11.5 g; Net Carbs: 6.5 g; Fat: 5 g; Protein: 5 g; Fibre: 5 g

SUPPER

TRADITIONAL SHAKSHUKA

4 servings
Net carbs: 12 g per serving

Ingredients

- 45 ml (3 tbsp) olive oil
- 1 onion, thinly sliced
- 1 red pepper, deseeded and sliced
- 1–2 red chillies, deseeded and thinly sliced (optional)
- 3 garlic cloves, finely chopped
- 2 tsp ground cumin
- 2 tbsp smoked paprika (not the hot spicy type)
- 1 x 400 g (14 oz) tin chopped tomatoes
- Large handful of chopped fresh coriander
- 8 medium free-range eggs

Method

- Heat the olive oil gently in a large cast-iron skillet over a low heat.
- Add the onion, red pepper and chillies and cook until a little charred – this should take about 6 minutes over a low heat.
- Add the garlic, cumin and paprika and cook for just 1 minute – do not burn the spices.

- Add the chopped tomatoes and simmer for 10 minutes, then season with salt and pepper to taste.
- Add half the coriander.
- Crack an egg into a small dish. Using a large spoon, make a well in the tomato mixture near the edge of the pan. Place the egg in the well, then repeat for all the eggs. The yolks should be exposed and not covered by the tomato mixture.
- Cover the pan with a lid and cook over a low heat until the whites are firm but the yolks still runny, which takes about 8 minutes.
- Garnish with the remaining coriander and serve.

Macronutrients per serving

- Calories: 287; Total Carbs: 13.25 g; Net Carbs: 12 g; Fat: 18 g; Protein: 11.2 g; Fibre: 1.25 g

GREEN SHAKSHUKA

4 servings
Net carbs: 13 g per serving

Ingredients

- 45 ml (3 tbsp) olive oil
- 6 spring onions, thinly sliced (including stems)
- 1–2 green chillies, deseeded and thinly sliced (optional)
- 3 garlic cloves, finely chopped
- 1 tsp ground cumin
- 1 tsp ground coriander
- ½ tsp fresh or dried oregano
- 200 g (about 3 cups/7 oz) kale, chopped (remove the stems if they are too agricultural for you!)
- Handful of chopped fresh curly parsley
- 125 ml (½ cup) vegetable stock
- 6 medium free-range eggs
- 50 g (⅓ cup) feta cheese, crumbled
- Handful of fresh dill
- Sea salt and black pepper

Method

- Heat the olive oil in a large cast-iron skillet over a low heat.
- Add the spring onions and chillies and cook until a little charred – this should take about 6 minutes.
- Add the garlic, cumin, coriander and oregano and cook for just 1 minute as you do not want to overcook the spices.
- Add the chopped kale and season with salt and pepper to taste.
- Cook until the kale starts to wilt, which takes about 5 minutes, or for longer if you do not like kale al dente.
- Add the chopped parsley and stock and cook for about 5 minutes until the liquid has almost evaporated.
- Crack an egg into a small dish. Using a large spoon, make a well in the kale mixture near the edge of the pan and place the egg in the well. Repeat for all the eggs. The yolks should be exposed and not covered by the kale mixture.
- Cover the pan with a lid and cook over a low heat until the whites are firm, but the yolks are still runny; this will take about 8 minutes. When the top of the egg goes white, it is usually no longer runny.
- Garnish with the crumbled feta cheese and dill and serve.

Macronutrients per serving

- Calories: 320; Total Carbs: 15.25 g; Net Carbs: 13 g; Fat: 21 g; Protein: 13 g; Fibre: 2.25 g

SHEPHERD'S PIE

4 servings
Net carbs: 8.5 g per serving

Ingredients

- 30 ml (2 tbsp) extra virgin cold pressed olive oil
- 500 g (1 lb 2 oz) minced lamb
- 1 medium white onion, finely chopped
- 2 carrots, finely diced
- 2 sticks of celery, finely diced

- 1 garlic clove, diced
- 1 tbsp tomato purée
- 500 ml (2 cups) beef stock or bone broth
- 2 bay leaves, broken in half
- Few sprigs of fresh thyme, roughly chopped
- Fresh rosemary, roughly chopped
- Cauliflower mashed 'potatoes' (see page 241)
- 50 g (2 oz/⅔ cup) grated Cheddar cheese
- Sea salt and black pepper

Method

- Heat the olive oil in a large pan over a medium heat. Add the mince and brown, ensuring all lumps are broken up. This will take a few minutes. Remove from the pan and set to one side.
- Add the onion, carrots and celery to the pan and cook over a low heat until tender, about 15–20 minutes.
- Add the garlic and tomato purée and cook for a few minutes.
- Return the mince to the pan and stir in.
- Add the stock, bay leaves and thyme and season with salt and pepper.
- Cover with a lid and simmer for 30 minutes, adding a little more stock if it looks like the mixture is drying out.
- Preheat the oven to 200°C/400°F/Gas mark 6.
- Tip the mince mixture into a large casserole dish and top with the cauliflower mashed 'potatoes'.
- Top with the grated Cheddar cheese and bake in the oven for 25–30 minutes until golden on top.
- Serve alone or with buttered leeks (see page 239).

Macronutrients per serving

- Calories: 468; Total Carbs: 17.5 g; Net Carbs: 8.5 g; Fat: 33 g; Protein: 29 g; Fibre: 9 g

CHRISTINE'S COTTAGE PIE

6 servings
Net carbs: 8.5 g per serving

Ingredients

- 15 ml (1 tbsp) extra virgin cold pressed olive oil
- 1 medium white onion, finely chopped
- 1 large carrot, finely diced
- 2 sticks of celery, finely diced
- 750 g (1½ lb) minced beef
- 1 tbsp tomato purée
- 500 ml (2 cups) rich beef stock
- Sea salt and black pepper
- Cauliflower 'potatoes' (see page 241)
- 50 g (2 oz/⅔ cup) grated Cheddar cheese

Method

- Preheat the oven to 140°C/275°F/Gas mark 1.
- Heat the oil in a large cast-iron casserole dish over a low heat.
- Add the onion, carrot and celery to the casserole and cook until soft, about 2–3 minutes.
- Add the minced beef to casserole and brown, ensuring all lumps are broken up; this will take up to 10 minutes.
- Add the tomato purée and cook for 2–3 minutes, then add the beef stock and season well with salt and pepper.
- Transfer to the oven and cook for 1½ hours.
- Allow to cool before topping with the cauliflower mashed 'potatoes' and grated cheese.
- Return to the oven for a further 30 minutes until golden and crispy on top.
- Serve alone or with haricots verts (see page 247).

Macronutrients per serving

- Calories: 461; Total Carbs: 17.5 g; Net Carbs: 8.5 g; Fat: 33 g; Protein: 29 g; Fibre: 9 g

SASFI'S CREAMY GARLIC PRAWNS

4 servings
Net carbs: 4.5 g per serving

Ingredients

- 300 g (11 oz) asparagus spears
- 3 garlic cloves, thinly sliced
- 15 ml (1 tbsp) olive oil
- 30 ml (2 tbsp) coconut oil
- 400 g (14 oz) uncooked peeled king prawns
- 1 medium tomato, chopped
- 125 ml (½ cup) cream
- 70 g (2½ oz) grated Parmesan cheese
- Large handful of torn basil
- Sea salt and black pepper

Method

- Preheat the oven to 180°C/350°F/Gas mark 4.
- Put the asparagus spears into a medium-sized baking tray, sprinkle with a third of the garlic and drizzle with olive oil. Bake in the oven for 10 minutes.
- Add the half the coconut oil to a skillet and place over a medium heat.
- Add the prawns to the pan and season with salt and pepper. Cook for a few minutes, stirring and turning until the prawns are cooked.
- Remove the prawns from the pan and set aside.
- Add the remaining coconut oil to the pan (if necessary) and add the remaining garlic; cook for 2 minutes without browning.
- Add the chopped tomatoes and cook for 2 more minutes, then add the cream and Parmesan and gently simmer for 1 minute. Season with black pepper.
- Return the prawns to the pan and heat everything together for a few minutes.
- Garnish with torn basil and serve in bowls with the asparagus on the side.

Macronutrients per serving

- Calories: 416; Total Carbs: 6.5 g; Net Carbs: 4.5 g;
  Fat: 34 g; Protein: 25 g; Fibre: 2 g

SALMON FILLETS WITH CHIMICHURRI SAUCE

1 serving
Net carbs: 1 g per serving

Ingredients

- 1 x 130 g (4½ oz) salmon fillet
- Ghee, butter or olive oil
- Sea salt and black pepper
- Lime or lemon wedges, to serve
- Chimichurri sauce (see page 248)
- Braised fennel (see page 243)

Method

- Preheat the oven to 180°C/350°F/Gas mark 4.
- Pat the salmon fillet dry with kitchen paper and season with salt and pepper.
- Rub the skin with ghee, butter or olive oil.
- Place an ovenproof frying pan or skillet over a medium heat; when hot place the salmon in the pan, skin side down, and cook for a few minutes until the skin is crispy.
- Transfer the pan to the oven and bake for 5 minutes.
- Serve with lemon or lime wedges, chimichurri sauce and braised fennel.

Macronutrients per serving

- Calories: 281; Total Carbs: 1 g; Net Carbs: 1 g;
  Fat: 21 g; Protein: 23 g; Fibre: 0 g

KAY AND MARCELLO'S BOLOGNESE SAUCE WITH COURGETTI

8 servings
Net carbs: 14 g per serving

Ingredients

- 15 ml (1 tbsp) olive oil
- 3 bay leaves, broken in half
- 1 large white onion, very finely chopped
- 4 garlic cloves, finely chopped
- 1.5 kg (3 lb 4 oz) minced beef
- 170 g (6 oz) tomato purée
- 3 x 400 g (14 oz) tins chopped tomatoes (ensure unsweetened)
- Large handful of finely chopped basil
- 1 beef stock cube
- 250 ml (1 cup) red wine
- Sea salt and black pepper

Method

- Chop the large onion finely in a blender.
- Pass the tinned tomatoes through a mouli grater.
- Heat the olive oil in a large cast-iron pan over a medium heat.
- Add the bay leaves and onion and stir and sweat for 5–7 minutes. The onion should be softened, but not browned.
- Add the garlic and cook for a further 3 minutes.
- Add the minced beef, stirring until it is broken up and browned.
- Stir in the tomato purée and cook over a low heat for a few minutes.
- Pass the tinned tomatoes through a mouli grater, then add to the pan. Add ½ cup of water, from rinsing the tins.
- Add the chopped basil, beef stock cube and red wine and season with salt and pepper to taste
- Cook over a low heat for 25 minutes, adding ½ cup of water, if necessary, to achieve a mildly soupy consistency.
- Serve on a bed of courgetti (see page 240).

Macronutrients per serving

- Calories: 588; Total Carbs: 16 g; Net Carbs: 14 g; Fat: 41 g; Protein: 37 g; Fibre: 2 g

CHICKEN TIKKA

2 servings
Net carbs: 5 g per serving

Ingredients

- ½ tsp salt
- ½ tsp ground black pepper
- 1 tsp ground cumin
- 1 tsp garam masala
- 1 tsp ground asafoetida
- 1 tsp ground fenugreek
- 1 tsp ground turmeric
- ½–2 tsp hot chilli powder, to taste
- 1 tsp green cardamom pods
- 1 tsp mustard seeds
- 1 tsp coriander seeds
- 1 tsp cumin seeds
- 45 ml (3 tbsp) olive oil
- 250 g (¾ cup) full-fat Greek yoghurt
- 2 x 130g (4½ oz) chicken breasts, cut into even-sized chunks (about 6 per chicken breast)
- Juice of 1 lemon

Method

- Mix the salt, pepper, ground cumin, garam masala, asafoetida, fenugreek, turmeric and chilli powder together. This is your powdered mix.
- Store in a sealed glass jar and label.
- Grind the cardamom pods, mustard seeds, coriander seeds and cumin seeds using a pestle and mortar to a fine powder, removing and discarding the cardamom husks. This is your dry mix.

- Store in a sealed glass jar and label.
- Place the olive oil and yoghurt into a bowl and gently stir together.
- Add 3 heaped teaspoons of the powdered mix (see above), then add 1 teaspoon of the dry mix (see above). Stir until combined.
- Add the chicken breast pieces and stir to coat, then cover and leave to marinate in the fridge for a few hours.
- Heat the grill (or set up a barbecue) to a hight heat.
- Thread the chicken onto skewers. (Note: the turmeric will stain your hands and everything else!)
- Cook under the grill or on the barbecue for several minutes, turning regularly. Regular splashes of lemon juice will help the flavour.
- Serve with mint yoghurt, onion raita and Turkish salad (see pages 251, 221 and 222).

Macronutrients per serving

- Calories: 575; Total Carbs: 5 g; Net Carbs: 5 g; Fat: 33.5 g; Protein: 62 g; Fibre: 0 g

BAKED COD WITH CHORIZO TOPPING

4 servings
Net carbs: 2.5 g per serving

Ingredients

- 100 g (3½ oz) Spanish chorizo, shredded to crumbs in blender
- 100 g (3½ oz) Parmesan cheese, finely grated in blender
- 18 g (3 tbsp) almond flour
- 14 g (½ oz/1 tbsp) butter
- Zest and juice of ½ lime
- 4 x 220 g (8 oz) skinned cod fillets
- Sea salt and black pepper
- Lime wedges, to serve

Method

- Preheat the oven to 200°C/400°F/Gas mark 6 and line a baking tray with foil.
- Put the chorizo, Parmesan cheese and almond flour into a bowl.
- Add the butter and season with salt and pepper.
- Use your fingers to blend together until the texture is like crumbs.
- Add the lime zest and juice and stir together.
- Place the fish on the lined baking tray, then spoon the mixture over the fish and press down.
- Bake in the oven for 10 minutes until the top is golden.
- Remove from oven and leave to rest in tray for 10 minutes.
- Serve with lime wedges, accompanied by buttered leeks, cauliflower mashed 'potatoes' or haricots verts (see pages 239, 241 and 247)

Macronutrients per serving

- Calories: 403; Total Carbs: 3 g; Net Carbs: 2.5 g; Fat: 21.5 g; Protein: 48 g; Fibre: 0.5 g

Variation

- This topping works with haddock, pollock, hake, grouper or any white fish.
- If you don't like lime, the recipe works perfectly well without it.

GREEK MARINATED CHICKEN

4 servings
Net carbs: 1 g per serving

Ingredients

- 4 garlic cloves, finely grated
- Juice of 1 lemon
- 80 ml (5 tbsp/⅓ cup) olive oil
- 60 ml (3 tbsp/¼ cup) red wine vinegar
- 1 tsp dried oregano

- 2 tsp dried thyme
- 4 boneless, skinless chicken breasts
- Sea salt and black pepper

Method

- Mix the garlic, lemon juice, olive oil, red wine vinegar, herbs and seasoning in a bowl.
- Place the chicken breasts in a dish.
- Pour the marinade over the chicken breasts, ensuring all the chicken is coated.
- Cover and place in the fridge for 1 hour.
- Heat a grill to high.
- Grill the chicken breasts for 15–20 minutes, turning the chicken halfway through cooking.
- Allow to rest for a few minutes before serving.
- Serve with a Greek salad (see page 223).

Macronutrients per serving

- Calories: 384; Total Carbs: 1 g; Net Carbs: 1 g; Fat: 21 g; Protein: 35 g; Fibre: 0 g

VEGETABLES

BUTTERED LEEKS

4 servings
Net carbs: 2 g per serving

Ingredients

- 1 kg (2 lb 2 oz) leeks, washed and thinly sliced diagonally
- 45 g (3 tbsp) butter
- Fresh thyme sprigs, leaves picked
- Sea salt and black pepper

Method

- Melt most of the butter in a large lidded saucepan over a medium heat.
- Add the leeks and season with salt and pepper.
- Stir to coat all the leeks with butter, then turn the heat down.
- Cover and cook until the leeks are soft, about 15 minutes, stirring once or twice. Do not allow the leeks to brown.
- Add the remaining butter and garnish with the thyme leaves.
- Serve as a side dish with fish or cottage pie (see page 231).

Macronutrients per serving

- Calories: 58; Total Carbs: 7 g; Net Carbs: 2 g;
  Fat: 1.3 g; Protein: 4 g; Fibre: 5 g

COURGETTI

4 servings
Net carbs: 9 g per serving

Ingredients

- 800 g (1 lb 12 oz/4 medium) fresh, firm courgettes
- 15 g (1 tbsp) butter
- Sea salt and black pepper

Method

- Prepare the courgettes with a spiraliser or julienne peeler or, if you have neither, make long strips with a vegetable peeler. You may wish to cut the lengths in half.
- Melt the butter gently in a large frying pan over a low heat.
- Add the courgettes strips and season with salt and pepper.
- Stir with a wooden spoon to coat the courgette strips in the butter.
- Cook for 1–3 minutes over a low heat; you want to warm the courgetti, not wilt it.
- Use as an alternative to pasta, served with bolognese or other sauces.

Macronutrients per serving

- Calories: 83; Total Carbs: 10 g; Net Carbs: 9 g; Fat: 3 g; Protein: 4 g; Fibre: 1 g

Variation

- Courgetti can also be eaten raw in salads: toss with lemon juice to soften and add finely chopped mint and finely chopped red chilli (optional).

CAULIFLOWER MASHED 'POTATOES'

4 servings
Net carbs: 4 g per serving

Ingredients

- 900 g (2 lb/or 1 medium) cauliflower without leaves, chopped into florets or chunks
- 50 ml (4 tbsp) double cream (optional; use for a smooth mash)
- Sea salt

Method

- Steam the cauliflower florets until tender: 5–6 minutes for a firm mash with a lumpy texture; 7–10 minutes for a creamier, smoother mash.
- Let the cauliflower stand for a few minutes in the steamer basket; it will lose steam and the mash will be less watery.
- Tip the cauliflower into a bowl and season with salt and pepper.
- Add the cream, if using, then use a hand potato masher to break up the cauliflower into small grain-like pieces, or continue to a smooth consistency, whichever you prefer. A food blender will help if you like it smooth.
- Serve as a substitute for mashed potatoes.

Macronutrients per serving

- Calories: 106; Total Carbs: 12 g; Net Carbs: 4 g; Fat: 6 g; Protein: 8 g; Fibre: 8 g

Variations

- Add 4 whole peeled garlic cloves to the cauliflower in the steamer and mash together.
- Add freshly chopped parsley, thyme, or rosemary or coriander, just before mashing.
- Add 30 g (1 oz/⅓ cup) grated cheese such as Parmesan, Cheddar or shredded Reblochon, just before mashing.

CELERIAC MASH

6 servings
Net carbs: 5 g per serving

Ingredients

- 1 medium whole celeriac, peeled and cut into, smallish, 2–3 cm (1 inch) cubes
- 50 g (2 oz/3½ tbsp) butter
- Sea salt and black pepper

Method

- Place the celeriac in a steamer and cook for about 15 minutes until soft.
- Tip the water out of the saucepan and add the celeriac to the dry pan.
- Add the butter and season with salt and pepper.
- Mash by hand or purée in a blender, depending on how smooth you like it. This mash is better left slightly lumpy; it can disappoint if you like a smooth mash.
- Serve with most meat dishes. It has a nutty flavour.

Macronutrients per serving

- Calories: 90; Total Carbs: 9.5 g; Net Carbs: 5 g; Fat: 6 g; Protein: 2 g; Fibre: 4.5 g

Variations

- Add grated horseradish for a bit of a kick.
- Add chopped herbs such as thyme leaves or rosemary.
- If you like it creamy and smooth, add a dollop of double cream as you are mashing.

BRAISED FENNEL

Serves 4
Net carbs: 16.5 g per serving

Ingredients

- 30 g (2 tbsp) butter
- 2 fennel bulbs, cut into quarters or eighths (save the top fronds to garnish)
- 2 garlic cloves, chopped
- 2 tsp chopped fresh rosemary
- 250 ml (1 cup) vegetable stock
- Zest and juice of 1 unwaxed lemon
- Sea salt and black pepper

Method

- Heat the butter in a cast-iron saucepan with a lid, large enough to fit all the fennel in a single layer (alternatively you can brown them in batches).
- Add the fennel pieces and brown over a medium heat on both sides; this will take about 1–2 minutes per side. Remove from the pan and set aside.
- Add the garlic and cook over a low heat until it is softened but not browned.
- Add the rosemary and vegetable stock and season with salt and pepper.
- Stir, scraping up the bits of caramelised fennel into the liquid, then return the fennel to the pan.
- Bring almost to the boil, cover and reduce the heat to low. Simmer for 40–50 minutes until the fennel is tender. If you prefer your vegetables al dente, reduce the simmering time to taste.
- Add the lemon zest and juice and remove from the pan.
- Garnish with fennel fronds and serve with salmon fillets (see page 233).

Macronutrients per serving

- Calories: 154; Total Carbs: 29 g; Net Carbs: 16.5 g; Fat: 2.5 g; Protein: 4 g; Fibre: 12.5 g

GARLIC MUSHROOMS

Serves 2
Net carbs: 5 g per serving

Ingredients

- 30 ml (2 tbsp) extra virgin olive oil
- 15 g (1 tbsp) butter
- 1 white onion, finely chopped
- 4 garlic cloves, finely chopped
- 300 g (10 oz) mushrooms, sliced
- 1 tsp finely chopped fresh thyme leaves
- 1 tsp finely chopped flat leaf parsley
- Chilli flakes (optional)
- Sea salt and black pepper

Method

- Gently heat the oil and butter in a skillet or cast-iron pan.
- Add the onion and cook until softened but not browned, about 5 minutes.
- Add the garlic and cook gently for a further 2–3 minutes. Do not brown.
- Add the mushrooms and cook gently over a low heat for 10–15 minutes until soft, stirring occasionally.
- Add the thyme and parsley (reserve some for garnish) and then add the chilli flakes, if using.
- Season to taste with salt and pepper, then garnish with the reserved parsley and serve warm.
- Can be eaten on its own or with steak.

Macronutrients per serving

- Calories: 220; Total Carbs: 7.5 g; Net Carbs: 5 g; Fat: 20 g; Protein:7.5 g; Fibre: 2.5 g

ROAST VEGETABLES

4 servings
Net carbs: 12 g per serving

Ingredients

- 5 garlic cloves, peeled but left whole
- 2 white onions, cut into eighths
- 1 cauliflower, cut into small florets
- 1 green pepper, cut into eighths
- Handful of green beans
- 10 cherry tomatoes on the vine
- 1–2 tsp dried oregano
- 1 tbsp olive oil
- Sea salt and black pepper
- 1–2 tsp chilli flakes

Method

- Preheat the oven to 200°C/400°F/Gas mark 6.
- Put the garlic, onions, cauliflower and green pepper in a large, shallow roasting pan and mix up.
- Add the green beans and cherry tomatoes in a layer on the top.
- Sprinkle the oregano liberally over the vegetables and drizzle with the olive oil.
- Season with salt and pepper and add the chilli flakes, to taste.
- Place in the oven and roast for 40–45 minutes, stirring halfway through the cooking time.
- Serve with roast meats, roast chicken breast, chops, steak or salmon fillet.

Macronutrients per serving

- Calories: 98; Total Carbs: 18 g; Net Carbs: 12 g; Fat: 0 g; Protein: 4.5 g; Fibre: 6 g

ROAST BROCCOLI

4 servings
Net carbs: 5 g per serving

Ingredients

- 680 g (1½ lb) broccoli florets
- 30 ml (2 tbsp) olive oil
- Juice of ½ lemon
- Sea salt and black pepper

Method

- Preheat the oven to 220°C/425°F/Gas mark 7 and line a roasting tray with foil (it is much easier to clean after).
- Toss the broccoli florets, lemon juice and olive oil in a bowl.
- Season with salt and pepper.
- Arrange the florets in an even layer in the roasting tray.
- Roast in the oven for 18–22 minutes until lightly toasted, stirring once halfway through the cooking time.
- This goes with most main courses.

Macronutrients per serving

- Calories: 109; Total Carbs: 10 g; Net Carbs: 5 g; Fat: 6.5 g; Protein: 5.5 g; Fibre: 5 g

Variations

- Sprinkle with red chilli flakes.
- Add grated garlic to the florets at the same time as the lemon juice.

HARICOTS VERTS

4 servings
Net carbs: 3.5 g per serving

Ingredients

- 500 g (1 lb 2 oz) haricots verts or thin green beans, trimmed
- 45 g (3 tbsp) butter
- 1 small red onion, finely chopped
- 2 tbsp chopped fresh parsley
- 2 tbsp chopped fresh thyme leaves
- 2 tbsp chopped fresh basil
- Sea salt and black pepper
- Lemon wedges, to serve

Method

- Blanch the beans in boiling water for 2 minutes.
- Meanwhile, prepare a large bowl with iced water.
- Drain the beans and plunge them into the iced water (this stops them cooking and helps them retain their colour).
- Drain the beans and pat dry with kitchen paper or leave on a wire rack until dry.
- In a frying pan, melt the butter and cook the onion in a single layer until translucent but not browned, about 3–4 minutes.
- Add the beans and sauté for 2–3 minutes.
- Add all the herbs and toss to blend the beans and herbs.
- Cook for a further 1–2 minutes.
- Serve with meat and fish dishes with a wedge of lemon.

Macronutrients per serving

- Calories: 77; Total Carbs: 7 g; Net Carbs: 3.5 g; Fat: 5 g; Protein: 2.5 g; Fibre: 4.5 g

CONDIMENTS

CHIMICHURRI

Serves 4–6
Net carbs: 1 g per serving

Ingredients

- 3 handfuls of finely chopped flat leaf parsley, leaves only
- 2 sprigs of finely chopped thyme leaves
- 2 spring onions, finely chopped
- 4 garlic cloves, very finely chopped
- 1½ tbsp chilli flakes
- 180 ml (¾ cup) organic apple cider vinegar
- Juice of 1 lemon
- 90 ml (6 tbsp) extra virgin cold pressed olive oil
- Sea salt and black pepper

Method

- You can use a food processor to prepare the ingredients if you prefer.
- Place the herbs, spring onions and garlic in a small bowl and mix together.
- Stir in the chilli flakes, vinegar, lemon juice and olive oil.
- Refrigerate for several hours.
- Chimichurri will keep for several days in the fridge.

Macronutrients per serving

- Calories: 126; Total Carbs: 1 g; Net Carbs: 0 g;
  Fat: 14 g; Protein: 0 g; Fibre: 0.2 g

KAY AND MARCELLO'S TOMATO SAUCE

Serves 12
Net carbs: 10 g per serving

Ingredients

- 8 x 400 g (14 oz) tins chopped tomatoes
- 2 medium white onions
- 4 garlic cloves
- Olive oil
- 3 bay leaves, broken in half
- ½ x 200 g (7 oz) tin tomato purée
- Handful of chopped fresh basil
- Handful of chopped fresh oregano
- 2 organic beef stock cubes, crumbled
- ½ glass of dry white wine
- Sea salt and black pepper

Method

- Pass tinned tomatoes through a stainless steel mouli grater.
- Chop the onions finely in blender or food processor.
- Chop the garlic finely in blender or food processor.
- Cover the base of a large heavy lidded pan with 1–2 ml of olive oil.
- Add the bay leaves, onions and garlic and sweat over a low heat for 2–3 minutes without browning them.
- Add the tinned tomatoes, tomato purée, basil and oregano.
- Add 3–5 cups of water until the sauce is the consistency of tomato soup.
- Season with salt and pepper to taste.
- Add the wine and crumbled beef stock cubes and stir in.
- Increase the heat until the sauce is simmering, then cover with the lid and simmer gently for 30 minutes.

- Use to make bolognese sauce, or add to green vegetables for a veg variation.

Macronutrients per serving

- Calories: 162; Total Carbs: 11.6 g; Net Carbs: 10.1 g; Fat: 12.5 g; Protein: 2.35 g; Fibre: 1.5 g

Note: This tomato sauce freezes well. You can split it into small proportions and then defrost as you need, which makes your dishes much quicker to prepare. Alternatively, you can divide the recipe by two or four and cook smaller amounts. It will keep in the fridge for a week.

VINAIGRETTE DRESSING

6 servings
Net carbs: 0 g per serving

Ingredients

- 1 tsp Dijon mustard
- 15 ml (1 tbsp) apple cider vinegar
- 1 tsp crushed sea salt
- Black pepper
- 90 ml (6 tbsp) extra virgin olive oil

Method

- Add the mustard to the vinegar and use a fork to mix thoroughly.
- Add the salt and black pepper to taste and mix with the vinegar.
- Add the olive oil.
- Pour into a lidded glass jar and shake vigorously.
- Use to dress your salad immediately before serving.

Macronutrients per serving

- Calories: 119; Total Carbs: 0 g; Net Carbs: 0 g; Fat: 14 g; Protein: 0 g; Fibre: 0 g

Variations

- You can use white wine, red wine or balsamic vinegar but not malt vinegar, which is too strong for salads. Keep the 6:1 proportion with the olive oil.
- Use any mustard of your choice, but very strong mustards may be a little overpowering.

MINT YOGHURT

6 servings
Net carbs: 3.7 g per serving

Ingredients

- 250 ml (1 cup) full-fat Greek yoghurt
- 2 tbsp mint sauce in vinegar
- 1 white onion, very finely chopped
- ½ tsp garam masala
- ½ tsp cayenne pepper
- Milk

Method

- Put the yoghurt into a bowl.
- Stir in the mint sauce.
- Add the chopped onion and spices and stir together.
- Add a little milk to achieve your desired consistency.

Macronutrients per serving

- Calories: 59; Total Carbs: 4 g; Net Carbs: 3.7 g; Fat: 4 g; Protein: 2 g; Fibre: 0.3 g

GLOSSARY

These are but wild and whirling words.

William Shakespeare, *Hamlet*

Aerobic metabolism: Aerobic metabolism refers to metabolism that uses oxygen, compared to anaerobic metabolism, which does not use oxygen. Fat metabolism is exclusively aerobic, and glucose metabolism can use either the aerobic or anaerobic pathway.

Agespan: The number of years that you live. It is also called your lifespan.

Anabolism: A type of metabolic process involving growth of new cells, maintenance of tissues and storage of energy for future use. It is a constructive type of metabolism.

Antioxidants: Antioxidants are chemicals found in foods. There are hundreds of foods that can act as antioxidants. They fight free radicals in your body.

Atheroma: Atheroma is the term used to describe a build-up of material in arteries. This is also known as plaque and can accumulate over time. Atheroma leads to heart attacks and strokes.

Atherosclerosis: Atherosclerosis is the condition caused by atheroma. See *atheroma*.

Adenosine diphosphate (ADP): Adenosine diphosphate is derived from ATP, when it has given up its energy.

Adenosine triphosphate (ATP): Adenosine triphosphate is the molecule that carries energy within cells.

Anaerobic metabolism: Anaerobic metabolism refers to metabolism that does not use oxygen, compared to aerobic metabolism, which uses oxygen.

Autophagy: Autophagy is a clean-up operation. It is the body's way of removing damaged cells and replacing these old cells with new, healthier ones. It is a process of recycling and cleaning. While autophagy happens naturally, it can be triggered by fasting and a keto diet. Autophagy is beneficial to your health.

Basal metabolic rate (BMR): Basal metabolic rate is the amount of energy your body uses to maintain vital functions such as your heart beating, breathing and staying warm.

Belly fat: is another term for *visceral fat*.

Blue Zones: Areas of the world where the inhabitants live the longest and demonstrate wellness for most of their lifetime. The people who live in Blue Zones have very low rates of long-term disease. They share commonalities of lifestyle.

Bioavailability: Bioavailability refers to the amount of a food or drug that is absorbed after eating. One hundred per cent bioavailability means that all the food or drug is absorbed and is able to have an active effect.

Body mass index (BMI): Body mass index is an indication of your body fat. It is based on your height and your weight. BMI tables give an indication as to whether you are underweight (<18.5), normal (18.5–24.9), overweight (25–29.9) or obese (>30). There are limitations to BMI as the formula cannot distinguish between fat and muscle. People who have a lot of muscle may appear to be overweight from their BMI. The unit of measurement is kg/m2.

Bowel: The bowel is part of your gut. It starts after the stomach and ends at your bottom. There is a small and large bowel, the small bowel being located before the large bowel. Its other names are intestine or colon.

Bug: A bug is an organism too small to be seen with the naked eye. They can only be seen with a microscope, hence their other names – microorganism and microbe. There are six major types, including bacteria, viruses and fungi. They are everywhere. They live in the soil, in rocks, in plants and animals. They live on our skin and in our guts. They have adapted to every environment in the world – snow fields, boiling hot springs and even the Antarctic. Microbial means relating to microbes (microorganisms/bugs).

Calorie density: The number of calories in a given weight of food. Foods have varying amounts of calories packed into them. For example, asparagus has 20 calories per 100 g and chocolate 500 calories per 100 g. Foods of low calorie density include vegetables, salads, fish, some fruit (particularly berries) and lean meat like chicken. Foods of high calorie density include fizzy drinks, crisps, condiments and sweets. See also *nutrient density*.

Calorie restriction: Calorie restriction is a long-term reduction of calories by 20–40 per cent, where meal frequency is maintained.

Carb: see *carbohydrate*.

Carbohydrate (CHO): one of the three macronutrients naturally found in food. Carbs are indigestible fibre (cellulose) or digestible (starches and sugars). The digestible are divided into quickly absorbed (high GI), or slowly absorbed (low GI). The quickly digested are either refined or super-refined.

Cardiovascular: A term for the circulatory system, which comprises the heart and blood vessels.

Catabolism: Catabolism is a process of energy provision for all cells. Cells break down stored carbohydrates and fat to release energy. It is a destructive type of metabolism.

CHO: See *carbohydrate*.

Cells: A cell is the basic unit of living things. All living things are made of cells. We are composed of 30 trillion cells. They are the factories of our bodies and make products that are used by surrounding cells. Cells are surrounded by walls and the entrances are tightly controlled by hormones such as insulin.

Cholesterol: Cholesterol is a fat, which is found in food and also made in your body. Eighty per cent comes from the liver, 20 per cent from diet.

Chromosome: A chromosome is a thread-like structure found in the centre (nucleus) of cells that carries unique genetic information, and are composed of DNA.

Circadian: Circadian refers to the natural cycle of biological rhythms, which recur on a 24-hour basis.

Circadian rhythm: The daily cycles of your mind, behaviour and body that follow a daily 24-hour cycle.

Colon: See *bowel*.

Correlation: See *causation*.

Cortisol: A hormone. It is called the 'fight or flight' hormone due to its pivotal role in the stress response, a vital part of our coping mechanisms. It has widespread effects on metabolism throughout the body.

Dementia: Dementia is an overall term for different types of conditions in which three main things happen: memory declines, communication difficulties develop and daily activities are adversely impacted. Alzheimer's is one of the commonest forms of dementia.

Diabetes: Diabetes is a disease that occurs when blood sugar is elevated. There is either a lack of insulin, as in type I diabetes or resistance to insulin as in type 2 diabetes.

Diseasespan: The number of years that you live with long-term disease before you die. People are developing long-term diseases at a younger age, living for a longer time with these diseases, and their diseasespan is lengthening.

Diurnal: This term applies to activity that is carried out during the day. Animals that are diurnal are active during the day and sleep at night. Processes in the body can show a diurnal rhythm, which means that they are more active during the day. Diurnal flowers are open during the day and closed at night.

DNA: Short for deoxyribonucleic acid, the building blocks of our genes. See *genes*.

EatSpan: EatSpan is the amount of time between your first meal of the day to your last meal.

Endocrine system: The endocrine system describes a system of glands that secrete hormones directly into the blood.

Environment: Human environment is a broad term and includes matter and conditions in the surroundings that impact on the development, action or survival of humans. It refers to all influences on us that are not genetically determined. It is a term used in the debate on nature versus nurture.

Epidemic: An epidemic is a disease that spreads over a wide area and affects many people at the same time. It is used to describe infections but is also widely used to describe the spread of obesity.

Fasting: Fasting is achieved by ingesting no food or calorific drinks for a period of 12 hours or more. Intermittent or periodic fasting means periods of fasting, interspersed with periods of normal eating. Here, we use the term 'fasting' to denote both intermittent and periodic fasting.

FastSpan: FastSpan is the amount of time spent fasting, between your last meal and the next meal.

Fat: Fat is one of the three main macronutrients along with carbohydrates and proteins.

Fat adaptation: The process by which we change our body from burning carbohydrate as a fuel to fat as a fuel.

Fat fuel inhibition (FFI): Fat fuel inhibition is our inability to switch from using carbohydrate as a fuel to using fat.

Fibre: Fibre is a form of carbohydrate that the body can't digest. It passes into the colon in an undigested form. The undigested fibre provides food for our gut bugs and bulk for poo. Fibre is essential for health.

Fizzy drinks: Fizzy drinks are also called carbonated sugary beverages, carbonated soda beverages, cola, pop, soda, soft drinks and soda pop. They may contain sugar or artificial sugar sweeteners or replacements.

Free radicals: These are chemicals that are highly unstable and reactive. Antioxidants stabilise free radicals and make them harmless.

Fructose: Fructose is a sugar, part of the carbohydrate group of foods. Fructose is naturally found in fruit, honey and most root vegetables. It is made into high fructose corn syrup.

Genes: Genes contain the instructions for how your body looks and works. Genes are present in all living things. Your genes are passed down from your parents. They are made from chemicals called DNA. If genes vary, we call this genetic variation.

Genetic: Genetics is the study of genes. See *genes*.

Ghrelin: Ghrelin is a hormone termed the hunger hormone and is responsible for making us feel hungry.

Glucagon: Glucagon is a hormone. Its actions are opposite to those of insulin. It signals to target cells to release glucose into the bloodstream.

Glucose: Glucose is sugar, part of the carbohydrate group of foods. Glucose is the simplest of sugars, with only one unit. When we talk about blood sugar, we mean blood glucose, which is the same thing.

Gluconeogenesis: Gluconeogenesis is the formation of glucose by the liver from fats or protein.

Glycogen: Glycogen is the storage form of glucose. It is composed of multiple glucose molecules linked together. Glycogen is found in the liver (30 per cent) and muscles (70 per cent). Animals also have glycogen and the plant equivalent is starch.

Glycolysis: Glycolysis is the breakdown of glucose to produce energy.

Glycogenolysis: Glycogenolysis is the breakdown of glycogen into glucose.

Glycogenesis: Glycogenesis is the formation of glycogen from glucose.

Glycaemic index (GI): The glycaemic index of food is the value given on the basis of how quickly the food raises blood sugar. Sugar is the reference food, with the highest glycaemic index, 100. The score is divided into high (>70), medium (56–69) and low (55).

Glycaemic load (GL): Glycaemic load combines the GI with the portion of food.

Gut: The gut is a long tube that runs from your mouth to your bottom. There are very tight defences between the inside of the gut and your body. The inside of your gut is considered to be outside your body.

Healthspan: The number of years that you live without developing long-term conditions. People who live to a ripe old age like 100 years have long healthspans. See diseasespan.

High fructose corn syrup (HFCS): High fructose corn syrup is a sweetener, ubiquitously found in processed foods and drinks. It is made from corn (maize) starch and is a very cheap food ingredient. There are different concentrations depending on the ratio of fructose and glucose, e.g. HFCS 55 contains 55 per cent fructose and 45 per cent glucose.

Homeostasis: Homeostasis means that our bodies are in equilibrium. The settings required are dynamic, responding to changes that we face. When the temperature changes, or we develop an infection, or our blood sugar goes up after a meal, our bodies adjust, to maintain a stable internal milieu. This is homeostasis. Hormones are largely responsible for controlling our homeostasis.

Hormones. Tiny chemical messenger (key) that travel in the blood to exert an effect on target cells, where there is a specific receptor (keyhole) for each hormone.

Hypertension: The medical term used to describe high blood pressure.

Hypo: See hypoglycaemia.

Hypoglycaemia: Hypoglycaemia occurs when your blood sugar drops below 4 mm/l. Hypoglycaemia happens if the body produces too much insulin after a sugary meal and blood sugar drops, an hour or two after eating. Symptoms of hypoglycaemia vary between individuals but include tiredness, hunger, trembling and sweating.

Inflammation: The body's response to an irritant. Inflammation can be localised, for example around a thorn in your finger, or generalised, for example the cytokine response to coronavirus. Inflammation is mounted by your immune system to protect you.

Inflammaging: Ageing itself is accompanied by low-level inflammation, a condition known as inflammaging.

Insulin: Insulin is a hormone. It allows sugars, fats and proteins into the cells. Insulin provides the key to allow energy to pass into the cell.

Insulin resistance: Insulin resistance means that the cells are resistant to the action of insulin and increasing amounts are needed to do the same job.

Insulin sensitivity: Insulin sensitivity is the opposite of insulin resistance.

Intestine: See *bowel.*

-itis: -itis at the end of a word implies inflammation. e.g. appendicitis is an inflamed appendix.

Ketones: Ketones are chemical substances that are made when fats are broken down for energy usage. They dissolve in water and cross into the brain, thus supplying it with energy. Ketones are also known as ketone bodies. Ketogenic means that the body is making ketones. You become ketogenic when you fast for prolonged periods, or follow a low-carbohydrate diet.

Ketogenic: see *ketones.*

Ketone bodies: see *ketones.*

Ketotic: Ketotic is an adjective of ketones, e.g. a ketotic state develops after fasting.

High-density lipoprotein (HDL): High-density lipoprotein is the 'good cholesterol'. HDL carries cholesterol in the blood. It returns low-density lipoprotein to the liver for processing. It helps to lower the risk of heart disease, heart attacks and stroke. Lipoproteins are produced in the liver.

Low-density lipoprotein (LDL): Low-density lipoprotein is the 'bad cholesterol' that collects in the wall of arteries. It is composed of fat and protein. LDL carries cholesterol in the blood. If your LDL is too high, you have a risk of developing heart disease, a heart attack or stroke. Lipoproteins are produced in the liver.

Lean: Lean means the absence of body fat. A lean person looks strong and healthy. If someone is lean, they have good muscle mass and low body fat. It is different to a thin person, who has low body fat but very little muscle.

Leptin: Leptin is a hormone. Leptin is produced by fat cells. It is called the satiety hormone and has a role in suppressing appetite.

Lifestyle choices: These are the choices that you make about how to live and behave. Lifestyle choices include what you eat and drink, whether you exercise or not, how you manage stress, whether you smoke or not and whether you take drugs. Lifestyle choices have a major impact on both your current and future health.

Lipid: Lipid is another term for fat.

Macronutrients: A macronutrient is a type of food required in large amounts in the diet. We typically refer to carbohydrates, fats and proteins as macronutrients. Water is usually considered to be a macronutrient, although it provides no energy.

Metabolic: The adjective relating to the metabolism of a living thing. See *metabolism*.

Metabolic syndrome: A condition where the chemical milieu of the body deteriorates, heralding the development of serious disease. Five factors develop: high blood pressure, high blood sugar, visceral fat, high triglyceride levels and low levels of good cholesterol or HDL. The presence of three or more of these factors means that you have metabolic syndrome.

Metabolically obese normal weight (MONW): This term refers to people who are defined as normal weight but show abnormalities of metabolism similar to obese people, with insulin resistance. People in this group have a greater risk of developing metabolic syndrome, diabetes and other long-term conditions.

Metabolism: Our metabolism is a group of chemical reactions, that keep us alive. The reactions involve changing food into energy or using energy. There are two main types of metabolic processes – anabolism (building) and catabolism (breakdown).

Microbe: See *bug*.

Microbial: See *bug*.

Microbiome: Microbiome is the term used for the bugs that coexist with you. The term is used interchangeably with *microbiota*. Strictly, *microbiome* refers to the genetic make-up of the bugs and *microbiota* refers to the bugs.

Microbiota: Microbiota is the term for the bugs that live with you. They are present in your gut (gut microbiota) and on your skin (skin microbiota).

Micronutrients: Micronutrients are foods needed in minuscule amounts but essential for health. Vitamins and minerals are examples of micronutrients.

Microorganism: See *bug*.

Mitochondria: Mitochondria are the powerhouses of the cell and make energy in the form of ATP. They are a type of organelle, lying within cells.

Mitophagy: Mitophagy is a form of autophagy that involves the mitochondria.

Monounsaturated fats (MUFA): Monounsaturated fats are fats with a double bond in their chemical structure.

Morbidity: Morbidity refers to having a disease. It is also used to denote the amount of disease in a population.

Mortality: Mortality refers to the causes of death on a large scale. For example, the falling mortality in Europe from coronavirus allowed relaxation of lockdown measures.

Muscle fibres: There are three main types of muscle fibres – slow twitch (ST), fast twitch I (FT-I) and fast twitch II (FT-II). Slow-twitch muscle fibres are resistant to fatigue and are our endurance muscle fibres.

Non-communicable diseases (NCDs): Non-communicable diseases are non-infectious diseases that cannot be spread from person to person, unlike an infectious disease, which spreads from person to person. Non-communicable diseases are responsible for 70 per cent of all deaths worldwide. The commonest non-communicable diseases are heart disease, stroke, cancer and chronic lung disease.

Nature: Nature refers to the physical world, including plants, animals and the landscape.

Nature versus nurture: An age-old argument in medicine. In this case, nature refers to our genes and nurture refers to our environment. The argument is between those who believe that nature determines our individuality and those who believe that nurture determines our individuality. Of course, it may be a bit of both.

Nucleus: The nucleus is the brain of the cell. It sits in the middle of the cell. The nucleus contains all the chromosomes and genes of that cell. It directs all the cell action.

Nurture: Nurture is the action or process of caring and protecting someone. It comes under the broad terms of 'environment'. See *nature versus nurture*.

Nutrient density: Nutrient density compares the number of nutrients to the calorific value of the weight of the food. The most nutrient-dense foods include kale, salmon, seaweed, garlic, shellfish, liver, eggs, blueberries and sardines. The least nutrient-dense food is sugar, with lots of calories and only one ingredient: sugar.

Obese: This is defined based on BMI (body mass index). Someone is obese if their BMI is over 30 kg/m2.

Obesity: see *obese*.

Organelles: Organelles are specialised structures within a living cell. Mitochondria are good examples of organelles; they are the powerhouse of cells.

Oxidative stress: An imbalance between chemicals that are unstable (free radicals) and chemicals (antioxidants) that are stable, which neutralise unstable chemicals. If free radicals overwhelm antioxidants, free radicals damage cells and this is oxidative stress. Oxidative stress plays a role in the development of many diseases.

Overweight: This is defined based on BMI (body mass index). Someone is overweight if their BMI is between 25 and 30 kg/m2.

Pandemic: A pandemic is the worldwide spread of a disease.

Polyphenol: Polyphenols are a beneficial plant chemical that help to keep you healthy and protect against various diseases. They are natural antioxidants. Polyphenols are found naturally, in plants such as red grapes and other fruits and vegetables as well as in green tea, herbs and spices.

Polyunsaturated fats (PUFA): Polyunsaturated fats contain more than one double bond in their chemical structure. The best known are omega-3 and omega-6 fatty acids. Your body can't make them, and they are critical for brain health. Polyunsaturated fats are found in oily fish including salmon, herring, mackerel and sardines. These essential fats are anti-inflammatory and healthy.

Prebiotics: Prebiotics are non-digestible fibre compounds, part of the carbohydrate macronutrient group, that pass through our digestive system into the colon. Prebiotics are essential food for our gut bugs, which ferment them in the colon.

Probiotics: Probiotics are live bacteria and yeasts that are good for you. They are found in fermented foods and pass into the intestine. Probiotics help to keep your gut bugs healthy.

Protein: Protein is one of the three main macronutrients along with carbohydrates and fats.

Receptor: A receptor is a part of tissue, or part of the cell wall, which binds specifically to a specific chemical, such as a hormone. Once a hormone binds to a receptor, the hormone can than transfer a message to the cell and this triggers a certain action.

Refined carbohydrates: See *carbohydrates*

Resveratrol: Resveratrol is a plant compound, part of a group called polyphenols.

Sarcopenia: The natural descent into frailty, characterised by loss of muscle and strength.

Saturated fats: A type of fat defined by their chemical structure. Saturated fats do not contain double bonds. Saturated fat is found in animals and plants including meat, butter, cheese and coconut oil.

Starvation: Starvation describes extreme forms of prolonged fasting – not intermittent fasting – which can result in degeneration or death. There is long-term deficiency of nutrients, resulting in harm.

Subcutaneous: Subcutaneous means under the skin.

Sucrose: Sucrose is table sugar. It is composed of one unit of glucose and one unit of fructose. Sucrose is a naturally occurring sugar, found in many plants – fruit, grains and vegetables. It is also added to many processed foods.

Super-refined carbohydrates: see *carbohydrates*.

Target cells: Cells that have receptors for a specific hormone (or other chemical). The term is also used to describe target tissue and target organs.

Telomeres: Telomeres are protective tips at the ends of chromosomes. They are a maker to life expectancy and are shortened by age and disease.

Thin: A thin person is someone who has low body fat and also has low muscle mass. They are not strong, and it is not as healthy as being *lean*. Lean is someone who has low body fat and also good muscle mass; they are strong and healthy.

Trans fats: These are killer saturated fats and must be avoided. They are also called partially hydrogenated fats.

Triglycerides: Triglycerides are fats composed of three fatty acids, hence the name. Most of our fat stores are composed of triglycerides. When they are transported in the blood, they are attached to the same carrier protein as cholesterol. Good fats, bad fats and in-between fats all contain triglycerides.

Unsaturated fats: Unsaturated fats have at least one double bond.

They include monounsaturated and polyunsaturated fats. They are the good boys of the fat family.

Vascular: A term that refers to blood vessels. For example, 'vascular disease' = blood vessel disease.

Visceral fat: Visceral fat, also called belly fat, is the unseen fat stored within the abdomen. It lies around your vital organs such as kidneys, liver, pancreas and intestines, and is very unhealthy.

Western Pattern Diet (WPD): The Western Pattern Diet is a modern-day style diet that is based on processed food, high-sugar foods and 'fast foods'. It increases the risk of long-term illness and is associated with abnormal metabolism and obesity. It is also called the Modern American Diet.

Whole grains: Whole grains mean that the entire grain is present: bran, germ and endosperm. Whole grains are not refined. They include oats, barley, wheat and rye.

World Health Organization (WHO): 'The World Health Organization is dedicated to the wellbeing of all people and guided by science, the World Health Organization leads and champions global efforts to give everyone, everywhere an equal chance to live a healthy life. Founded in 1948, WHO is the United Nations agency that connects nations, partners and people to promote health, keep the world safe and serve the vulnerable – so everyone, everywhere can attain the highest level of health.' WHO, 2021.

NOTES

INTRODUCTION

1 Ge L., Sadeghirad B., Ball G.D.C., et al. 'Comparison of dietary macro-nutrient patterns of 14 popular named dietary programmes for weight and cardiovascular risk factor reduction in adults: systematic review and network meta-analysis of randomised trials.' *BMJ*, 2020 Apr 1; 369:m696.

2 Wiebe N., Ye F., Crumley E.T., Bello A., et al. 'Temporal Associations Among Body Mass Index, Fasting Insulin, and Systemic Inflammation: A Systematic Review and Meta-analysis.' *JAMA Netw Open*. 2021; 4(3):e211263. doi:10.1001/jamanetworkopen.2021.1263

3 Mandini S., Conconi F., Mori E., et al. 'Walking and hypertension: greater reductions in subjects with higher baseline systolic blood pressure following six months of guided walking.' *PeerJ*. 2018; 6(5).

4 Wheeler M., Dunstan D., Ellis K., et al. 'Effect of morning exercise with or without breaks in prolonged sitting on blood pressure in older over-weight/ obese adults. Evidence for sex differences.' *Hypertension*. 2019; 73:859–867.

CHAPTER 1

1 Plomin R. 2018. *Blueprint*. Penguin.

2 Zhou Z., Macpherson J., Gray S.R., et al. 'Are people with metabolically healthy obesity really healthy? A prospective cohort study of 381,363 UK Biobank participants.' *Diabetologia*. 2021 Sep; 64(9):1963–1972. doi: 10.1007/s00125-021-05484-6. Epub 2021 Jun 10. PMID: 34109441.

3 Wallman, J. 2014. *Stuffocation: Living More with Less*. Penguin.

4 Manfredini R., Fabbian F., Cappadona R., et al. 'Daylight Saving Time and Acute Myocardial Infarction: A Meta-Analysis.' *J Clin Med*. 2019; 8(3):404. Published 2019 Mar 23. doi:10.3390/jcm8030404

5 Chattu V.K., Manzar M.D., Kumary S. et al. 'The Global Problem of Insufficient Sleep and Its Serious Public Health Implications.' *Healthcare*

(Basel). 2018 Dec 20; 7(1):1. doi: 10.3390/healthcare7010001. PMID: 30577441; PMCID: PMC6473877.

6 Moberly T. 'Doctors' early retirement has trebled since 2008.' *BMJ*, 2021; 373:n1594 doi:10.1136/bmj.n1594

7 Johnson R., Appel L., Brands M. 'Dietary sugar intake and cardiovascular health. A scientific statement from the American Heart Association.' *Circulation.* 2009; 120:1011–1020.

8 Lustig R. 2012. *Fat Chance.* Hudson Street Press.

CHAPTER 3

1 Rowling, J.K. 2014. *Harry Potter and the Philosopher's Stone.* New York, NY: Bloomsbury Childrens Books.

CHAPTER 4

1 *BBC News*, 1 October 2020.

2 Ray K.S., Singhania P.R. 'Glycemic and insulinemic responses to carbohydrate rich whole foods.' *J Food Sci Technol.* 2014; 51(2):347–352.

3 Younossi Z.M., Koenig A.B., Abdelatif D., et al. 'Global epidemiology of nonalcoholic fatty liver disease—meta-analytic assessment of prevalence, incidence, and outcomes.' *Hepatology.* 2016; 64(1):73–84. doi:10.1002/hep.28431

4 Shapiro, A., Mu, W., Roncal, C., et al. 'Fructose induced Leptin resistance induces obesity in high subsequent fat diets.' *Am J Comp Physiol* 2008 Nov:295(5):1370–5.

CHAPTER 5

1 Harcombe Z., Baker J.S., Cooper S.M., et al. 'Evidence from randomised controlled trials did not support the introduction of dietary fat guidelines in 1977 and 1983: a systematic review and meta-analysis.' *Open Heart* 2015; 2:e000196. doi: 10.1136/openhrt-2014-000196

2 Yerushalmy J., Hilleboe H.E. 'Fat in the diet and mortality from heart disease; a methodologic note.' *N Y State J Med.* 1957; 57:2343–2354.

3 Pelkman C., Fishell V., Maddox D. 'Effects of moderate-fat (from monounsaturated fat) and low-fat weight-loss diets on the serum lipid profile in overweight and obese men and women.' *The American Journal of Clinical Nutrition.* 2004; 79(2):204–212.

4 Esposito K., Marfella R., Ciotola M., et al. 'Effect of a Mediterranean-Style Diet on Endothelial Dysfunction and Markers of Vascular Inflammation in the Metabolic Syndrome: A Randomized Trial.' *JAMA.* 2004; 292(12):1440–1446.

5 Appel L.J., Sacks F.M., Carey V.J., et al. 'Effects of Protein,

Monounsaturated Fat, and Carbohydrate Intake on Blood Pressure and Serum Lipids: Results of the OmniHeart Randomized Trial.' *JAMA*. 2005; 294(19):2455–2464.

6   Van Dijk S., Feskens E., Bos M. et al. 'A saturated fatty acid–rich diet induces an obesity-linked proinflammatory gene expression profile in adipose tissue of subjects at risk of metabolic syndrome.' *The American Journal of Clinical Nutrition*. 2009; 90(6):1656–1664.

7   Simopoulos A. 'The importance of the 6/3 ratio in cardiovascular disease.' *Expl Biol and Med*. 2008; 233(6).

8   DiNicolantonio J.J., O'Keefe J.H. 'Importance of maintaining a low omega-6/omega-3 ratio for reducing inflammation.' *Open Heart*. 2018; 5(2)

9   Simopoulos A.P. 'An Increase in the Omega-6/Omega-3 Fatty Acid Ratio Increases the Risk for Obesity.' *Nutrients*. 2016; 8(3):128.

10 Simopoulos A.P. 'The importance of the ratio of omega-6/omega-3 essential fatty acids.' *Biomed Pharmacother*. 2002; 56(8):365–379.

11 Oddy W.H., de Klerk N.H., Kendall G.E., et al. 'Ratio of omega-6 to omega-3 fatty acids and childhood asthma.' *J Asthma*. 2004; 41(3):319–326.

12 Manson J.E., Bassuk S.S., Cook N.R., et al. 'VITAL study Vitamin D, Marine n-3 Fatty Acids, and Primary Prevention of Cardiovascular Disease Current Evidence.' *Circulation Research*. 2020; 126:112–128.

13 Bowden R.G., Wilson R.L., Beaujean A.A. 'LDL particle size and number compared with LDL cholesterol and risk categorization in end-stage renal disease patients.' *J Nephrol*. 2011; 24(6):771–777.

14 Ravnskov U., Diamond D.M., Hama R., et al. 'Lack of an association or an inverse association between low-density-lipoprotein cholesterol and mortality in the elderly: a systematic review.' *BMJ Open*. 2016 Jun 12; 6(6):e010401. doi: 10.1136/bmjopen-2015-010401. PMID: 27292972; PMCID: PMC4908872.

15 DiNicolantonio J.J. 'The cardiometabolic consequences of replacing saturated fats with carbohydrates or Ω-6 polyunsaturated fats: Do the dietary guidelines have it wrong?' *Open Heart*. 2014 Feb 8; 1(1).

CHAPTER 6

1   Cruz-Jentoft A., Sayer A. 'Sarcopoenia.' *The Lancet*. 2019; 393:2636–2646.

CHAPTER 7

1   Sender R., Fuchs S., Milo R. 'Revised Estimates for the Number of Human and Bacteria Cells in the Body.' *PLoS Biol* 2016; 14(8).

2   Lloyd-Price J., Abu-Ali G., Huttenhower C. 'The healthy human microbiome.' *Genome Medicine*. 2016; 8:51.

3 Dieterich W., Schink M., Zopf Y. 'Microbiota in the Gastrointestinal Tract.' *Med Sci* (Basel). 2018; 6(4):116.

4 Davenport E.R., Sanders J.G., Song S.J., et al. 'The human microbiome in evolution.' *BMC Biol.* 2017 Dec 27; 15(1):127.

5 Thursby E., Juge N. 'Introduction to the human gut microbiota.' *Biochem J.* 2017 May 16; 474(11):1823–1836.

6 Martens J.H., Barg H., Warren M.J., et al. 'Microbial production of vitamin B12.' *Appl Microbiol Biotechnol.* 2002;58(3):275–285.

7 LeBlanc J.G., Chain F., Martín R. et al. 'Beneficial effects on host energy metabolism of short-chain fatty acids and vitamins produced by commensal and probiotic bacteria.' *Microb Cell Fact.* 2017; 16(1):79.

8 Valdes A.M., Walter J., Segal E., et al. 'Role of the gut microbiota in nutrition and health.' *BMJ.* 2018; 361:k2179.

9 Carlucci C., Petrof E.O., Allen-Vercoe E. 'Fecal Microbiota-based Therapeutics for Recurrent Clostridium difficile Infection, Ulcerative Colitis and Obesity.' *EBioMedicine.* 2016; 13:37–45.

10 Tropini C., Earle K.A., Huang K.C., et al, The Gut Microbiome: Connecting Spatial Organization to Function. Cell Host Microbe. 2017; 21(4):433-442.

11 Dieterich W., Schink M., Zopf Y. 'Microbiota in the Gastrointestinal Tract.' *Med Sci* (Basel). 2018; 6(4):116.

12 Donaldson G.P., Lee M.S., Mazmanian S.K. 'Gut biogeography of the bacterial microbiota.' *Nat Rev Microbiol.* 2016; 14(1):20–32.

13 Sommer F., Anderson J., Bharti R., et al. 'The resilience of the intestinal microbiota influences health and disease.' *Nat Rev Microbiol* 2017; 15;630–638.

14 Kim S., Jazwinski S.M. 'The Gut Microbiota and Healthy Aging: A Mini-Review.' *Gerontology.* 2018; 64(6):513–520.

15 Gibbs R.A. 'The Human Genome Project changed everything.' *Nat Rev Genet* 2020; 21, 575–576.

16 Turnbaugh P., Ley R., Hamady M., et al. 'The Human Microbiome Project.' *Nature* 2007; 449;804–810.

17 Integrative HMP (iHMP) Research Network Consortium. 'The Integrative Human Microbiome Project.' *Nature.* 2019; 569(7758):641–648.

18 Bilen M., Dufour J.C., Lagier J.C., et al. 'The contribution of culturomics to the repertoire of isolated human bacterial and archaeal species.' *Microbiome.* 2018; 6(1):94.

19 Almeida A., A.L., Boland M., et al. 'A new genomic blueprint of the human gut microbiota.' *Nature.* 2019; 568:499–504.

20 Schloissnig S., Arumugam M., Sunagawa S., et al. 'Genomic variation landscape of the human gut microbiome.' *Nature.* 2013; 493(7430):45–50.

21 Tierney B., Yang Z., Luber J., et al. 'The Landscape of Genetic Content in the Gut and Oral Human Microbiome.' *Cell Host Microbe*. 2019; 26(2):283–295.

22 Rooks M.G., Garrett W.S. 'Gut microbiota, metabolites and host immunity.' *Nat Rev Immunol*. 2016; 16(6):341–352.

23 Rea K., Dinan T.G., Cryan J.F. 'Gut Microbiota: A Perspective for Psychiatrists.' *Neuropsychobiology*. 2020; 79(1):50–62.

24 Cryan J.F., de Wit H. 'The gut microbiome in psychopharmacology and psychiatry.' *Psychopharmacology* (Berl). 2019; 236(5):1407–1409.

25 Cryan J.F., O'Riordan K.J., Cowan C.S.M., et al. 'The Microbiota–Gut–Brain Axis.' *Physiol Rev*. 2019; 99(4):1877–2013.

26 Frost G., Sleeth M.L., Sahuri-Arisoylu M/, et al. 'The short-chain fatty acid acetate reduces appetite via a central homeostatic mechanism.' *Nat Commun*. 2014; (5):3611.

27 Moore T.J., Mattison D.R. 'Adult Utilization of Psychiatric Drugs and Differences by Sex, Age, and Race.' *JAMA Intern Med*. 2017 Feb 1; 177(2):274–275. Erratum in: *JAMA Intern Med*. 2017 Mar 1; 177(3):449.

28 Yano J., Yu K, Donaldson G., et al. 'Indigenous bacteria from the gut microbiota regulate host serotonin biosynthesis' [published correction appears in *Cell*. 2015 Sep 24; 163:258]. *Cell*. 2015; 161(2):264–276.

29 Agus A., Planchais J., Sokol H. 'Gut Microbiota Regulation of Tryptophan Metabolism in Health and Disease.' *Cell Host Microbe*. 2018; 23(6):716–724.

30 Carding S., Verbeke K., Vipond D.T., et al. 'Dysbiosis of the gut microbiota in disease.' *Microb Ecol Health Dis*. 2015; 26:26191.

31 Cani P.D. 'Human gut microbiome: hopes, threats and promises.' *Gut*. 2018; 67:1716–1725.

32 Castaner O., Goday A., Park Y.M., et al. 'The Gut Microbiome Profile in Obesity: A Systematic Review.' *Int J Endocrinol*. 2018; 2018:4095789.

33 Le Chatelier E., Nielsen T., Qin J., et al. 'Richness of human gut microbiome correlates with metabolic markers.' *Nature*. 2013; 500(7464):541–6.

34 McBurney M., Davis C., Fraser C.M., et al. 'Establishing What Constitutes a Healthy Human Gut Microbiome: State of the Science, Regulatory Considerations, and Future Directions.' *The Journal of Nutrition*. 2019; 149(11):1882–1895.

35 Asnicar F., Berry S.E., Valdes A.M., et al. 'Microbiome connections with host metabolism and habitual diet from 1,098 deeply phenotyped individuals.' *Nat Med*. 2021 Feb; 27(2):321–332.

36 Dao M.C., Everard A., Aron-Wisnewsky J., et al. 'Akkermansia muciniphila and improved metabolic health during a dietary intervention in

obesity: relationship with gut microbiome richness and ecology.' *Gut.* 2016; 65(3):426–436.

37 Remely M., Tesar I., Hippe B., et al. 'Gut microbiota composition correlates with changes in body fat content due to weight loss.' *Beneficial Microbes.* 2015; 6(4):431–439.

38 Özkul C., Yalınay M., Karakan T. 'Islamic fasting leads to an increased abundance of Akkermansia muciniphila and Bacteroides fragilis group: A preliminary study on intermittent fasting.' *Turk J Gastroenterol.* 2019; 30(12):1030–5.

39 Mohr A.E., Jäger R., Carpenter K.C., et al. 'The athletic gut microbiota.' *J Int Soc Sports Nutr.* 2020 May 12; 17(1):24.

40 Thaiss C.A., Zeevi D., Levy M., et al., 'A day in the life of the meta-organism: diurnal rhythms of the intestinal microbiome and its host.' *Gut Microbes.* 2015; 6(2):137–142.

41 Murakami M. and Tognini P. 'The Circadian Clock as an Essential Molecular Link Between Host Physiology and Microorganisms.' *Front. Cell. Infect. Microbiol.* 2020; 9:469.

42 Kaczmarek J.L., Thompson S.V., Holscher H.D. 'Complex interactions of circadian rhythms, eating behaviours, and the gastrointestinal microbiota and their potential impact on health.' *Nutr Rev.* 2017; 75(9):673–682.

43 Thaiss C.A., Zeevi D., Levy M., et al. 'Transkingdom control of micro-biota diurnal oscillations promotes metabolic homeostasis.' *Cell.* 2014; 159; 514–29.

CHAPTER 8

1 Cole G., Frautschy S. 'DHA may prevent age-related dementia.' *J Nutr.* 2010; 140(4):869–874.

2 Araújo J., Cai J., and Stevens J. 'Prevalence of optimum metabolic health in adults; National Survey 2009–16.' *J Metabolic Syndrome and Related Disorders.* 17(1);46–52.

3 Ruderman N.B., Schneider S.H. and Berchtold P. 'The "metabolically-obese," normal-weight individual.' *Am J Clin Nutr.* 1981; 34:1617–21.

4 Bradshaw P.T., Monda K.L. and Stevens J. 'Metabolic syndrome in healthy obese, overweight, and normal weight individuals: the Atherosclerosis Risk in Communities Study.' *Obesity* (Silver Spring). 2013; 21(1):203–209.

5 Ibid.

6 Zhou Z., Macpherson J., Gray S.R., et al. 'Are people with metabolically healthy obesity really healthy? A prospective cohort study of 381,363 UK Biobank participants.' *Diabetologia.* 2021 Sep; 64(9):1963–1972. doi: 10.1007/s00125-021-05484-6. Epub 2021 Jun 10. PMID: 34109441.

7   Rubenstein A.H. 'Obesity: a modern epidemic.' *Trans Am Clin Climatol Assoc.* 2005; 116:103–113.

8   Pi-Sunyer X. 'The medical risks of obesity.' *Postgrad Med.* 2009; 121(6):21–33.

9   An R., Yan H., Shi, X., et al. 'Childhood obesity and school absenteeism: a systematic review and meta-analysis.' *Obesity Reviews.* 2017; 18:1412–1424.

10 Fitzgerald S., Hirby A., Murphy A., et al. 'Obesity, diet quality and absenteeism in a working population.' *Public Health Nutrition.* 2016; 19(18):3287–3295.

11 Lee J., Lee J., Lee J. et al. 'Visceral fat obesity is highly associated with primary gout in a metabolically obese but normal weighted population: a case control study.' *Arthritis Res Ther.* 2015; 17:79.

12 Shen W., Punyanitya M., Chen J., et al. 'Waist circumference correlates with metabolic syndrome indicators better than percentage fat.' *Obesity* (Silver Spring). 2006; 14(4):727–736.

13 Kaur J. 'A comprehensive review on metabolic syndrome' [retracted in: *Cardiol Res Pract. 2019* Jan 31;2019:4301528]. *Cardiol Res Pract.* 2014; 2014: 943162.

14 Shen W., Punyanitya M., Chen J., et al. 'Waist circumference correlates with metabolic syndrome indicators better than percentage fat.' *Obesity* (Silver Spring). 2006; 14(4):727–736.

15 Flint A., Rexrode K., Hu F., et al. 'Body mass index, waist circumference, and risk of coronary heart disease: a prospective study among men and women.' *Obes Res Clin Pract.* 2010 Jul; 4(3):e171–e181.

16 Lee K.R., Seo M.H., Do Han K., et al. 'Waist circumference and risk of 23 site-specific cancers: a population-based cohort study of Korean adults.' *Br J Cancer.* 2018; 119:1018–1027.

17 Flegal K., Kit B., Orpana H., Graubard B. 'Association of all-cause mortality with overweight and obesity using standard body mass index categories: a systematic review and meta-analysis.' *JAMA.* 2013 Jan 2; 309(1):71–82.

18 Kenneth A., Schatzkin A., Harris T., et al. 'Overweight, Obesity, and Mortality in a Large Prospective Cohort of Persons 50 to 71 Years Old.' *N Engl J Med.* 2006; 355:763–778.

19 Arnlöv J., Sundström J., Ingelsson .E, et al. 'Impact of BMI and the metabolic syndrome on the risk of diabetes in middle-aged men.' *Diabetes Care.* 2011; 34(1):61–65.

20 Flint A., Rexrode K., Hu F., et al. 'Body mass index, waist circumference, and risk of coronary heart disease: a prospective study among men and women.' *Obes Res Clin Pract.* 2010 Jul; 4(3):e171–e181.

21 Lee K.R., Seo M.H., Do Han K., et al. 'Waist circumference and risk of

23 site-specific cancers: a population-based cohort study of Korean adults.' *Br J Cancer*. 2018; 119:1018–1027.

22 Krakauer N.Y., Krakauer J.C. 'A new body shape index predicts mortality hazard independently of body mass index.' *PLoS One*. 2012; 7(7):e39504. doi:10.1371/journal.pone.0039504

23 Aucouturier J., Meyer M., Thivel D. et al. 'Affect of Android to Gynoid fat ratio on Insulin Resistance in Obese Youth.' *Arch Pediatr Adolesc Med*. 2009 Sep; 163(9):826–31.

24 Aucouturier J, Meyer M, Thivel D et al. Arch Pediatr Adolesc Med. 2009 Sep; 163(9):826-31.

CHAPTER 9

1 Ge L., Sadeghirad B., Ball G.D.C., et al. 'Comparison of dietary macronutrient patterns of 14 popular named dietary programmes for weight and cardiovascular risk factor reduction in adults: systematic review and network meta-analysis of randomised trials.' *BMJ*. 2020; 369:m696.

2 Ibid.

3 Meerman R., Brown, A.J. 'When somebody loses weight where does the fat go?' *BMJ*. 2014; 349:g7257.

4 Janseen I., Heymsfield S.B., Wang Z. 'Skeletal muscle mass and distribution in 468 men and women aged 18–88 yr.' *J.App. Phys*. 2000; 89:81–88.

5 Osterberg K.L., Melby C.L. 'Effect of acute resistance exercise on post-exercise oxygen consumption and resting metabolic rate in young women' [published correction appears in. *Int J Sport Nutr Exerc Metab*. 2000 Sep; 10(3):360]. *Int J Sport Nutr Exerc Metab*. 2000; 10(1):71–81.

6 Melanson E.L., MacLean P.S., Hill J.O. 'Exercise improves fat metabolism in muscle but does not increase 24-h fat oxidation.' *Exerc Sport Sci Rev*. 2009; 37(2):93–101.

CHAPTER 10

1 Shapiro A., Mu W., Roncal C., et al. 'Fructose induced Leptin resistance induces obesity in high subsequent fat diets.' *Am J Comp Physiol*. 2008 Nov: 295(5):1370–5.

2 Thau L., Sharma S. 'Physiology, Cortisol.' [Updated 2020 Mar 24]. In: *StatPearls* [Internet]. Treasure Island (FL): StatPearls Publishing; 2020 Jan.

3 Ludwig D.S., Aronne L.J., Astrup A., et al. 'The carbohydrate-insulin model: a physiological perspective on the obesity pandemic.' *Am J Clin Nutr*. 2021 Sep 13; nqab270.

CHAPTER 11

1   Wooden J. and Jamison S. *Wooden: A Lifetime of Observations and Reflections On and Off the Court.* McGraw Hill. 1997.

CHAPTER 12

1   Heilbronn L.K., Smith S.R., Martin C.K., et al. 'Alternate-day fasting in nonobese subjects: effects on body weight, body composition, and energy metabolism.' *Am J Clin Nutr.* 2005; 81(1):69–73.

2   Hartman M., Veldhuis J., Johnson M. 'Augmented growth homone secretion, frequency and amplitude mediate enhanced GH secretion during a two day fast in normal men.' *J of Clin End Metab.* 1992; 74;(4) 757–765.

3   Johnson J.B., Summer W., Cutler R.G., et al. 'Alternate day calorie restriction improves clinical findings and reduces markers of oxidative stress and inflammation in overweight adults with moderate asthma' [published correction appears in *Free Radic Biol Med.* 2007 Nov 1;43(9):1348. Tellejohan, Richard [corrected to Telljohann, Richard]]. *Free Radic Biol Med.* 2007; 42(5):665–674.

4   Fung, J. (2016) *The Obesity Code: Unlocking the Secrets of Weight Loss.* Vancouver: Greystone Books.

CHAPTER 13

1   Belbin F.E., Hall G.J., Jackson A.B., et al. 'Plant circadian rhythms regulate the effectiveness of a glyphosate-based herbicide.' *Nature Communications.* 2019; 10(1).

2   Nobs S.P., Tuganbaev T., Elinav E. 'Microbiome diurnal rhythmicity and its impact on host physiology and disease risk.' *EMBO Rep.* 2019; 20(4):e47129.

3   Partch C.L., Green C.B., Takahashi J.S. 'Molecular architecture of the mammalian circadian clock.' *Trends Cell Biol.* 2014; 24(2):90–99.

4   Aschoff J. 'Spontanperiodik des Menschen bei Aussschulss aller Sietgeber.' *Naturwissenschaften.* 1962; 49:33–42.

5   Aschoff J. 'Exogenous and Endogenous Components in Circadian Rhythms'. *Cold Spring Harb Symp Quant Biol.* 1960; 25:11–28.

6   Panda S., Antoch M.P., Miller B.H., et al. 'Coordinated transcription of key pathways in the mouse by the circadian clock.' *Cell.* 2002; 109(3):307–20.

7   Foster R.G., Provencio I., Hudson D., et al. 'Circadian photoreception in the retinally degenerate mouse (rd/rd).' *J Comp Physiol A.* 1991; 169(1):39–50.

8   Freedman M.S., Lucas R.J., Soni B., et al. 'Regulation of mammalian

circadian behavior by non-rod, non-cone, ocular photoreceptors.' *Science.* 1999; 284(5413):502–4.

9 Lucas R.J., Freedman M.S., Muñoz M., et al. 'Regulation of the mammalian pineal by non-rod, non-cone, ocular photoreceptors.' *Science.* 1999; 284(5413):505–7.

10 Panda S., Sato T.K., Castrucci A.M., et al. 'Melanopsin (Opn4) requirement for normal light-induced circadian phase shifting.' *Science.* 2002; 298(5601):2213–6.

11 Ruby N.F., Brennan T.J., Xie X., et al. 'Role of melanopsin in circadian responses to light.' *Science.* 2002; 298(5601):2211–3.

12 Hattar S., Liao H.W., Takao M., et al. 'Melanopsin-containing retinal ganglion cells: architecture, projections, and intrinsic photosensitivity.' *Science.* 2002; 295(5557):1065–70.

13 Berson D.M., Dunn F.A., Takao M. 'Phototransduction by retinal ganglion cells that set the circadian clock.' *Science.* 2002; 295(5557):1070–3.

14 Emens J.S., Eastman C.I. 'Diagnosis and Treatment of Non-24-h Sleep-Wake Disorder in the Blind.' *Drugs.* 2017; 77(6):637–650.

15 Hatori M., Gronfier C., Van Gelder R.N., et al. 'Global rise of potential health hazards caused by blue light-induced circadian disruption in modern aging societies.' *NPJ Aging Mech Dis.* 2017; 16;(3):9.

16 Zhang Q., Chair S.Y., Lo S.H.S., et al. 'Association between shift work and obesity among nurses: A systematic review and meta-analysis.' *Int J Nurs Stud.* 2020; 112:103757.

17 Kecklund G., Axelsson J. 'Health consequences of shift work and insufficient sleep.' *BMJ.* 2016; 355:i5210.

18 Stenvers D.J., Scheer F.A.J.L., Schrauwen P., et al. 'Circadian clocks and insulin resistance.' *Nat Rev Endocrinol.* 2019 Feb; 15(2):75–89.

19 Flanagan A., Bechtold D.A., Pot G.K., et al. 'Chrono-nutrition: From molecular and neuronal mechanisms to human epidemiology and timed feeding patterns.' *J Neurochem.* 2021; 157(1):53–72.

20 Chang A.M., Duffy J.F., Buxton O.M., et al. 'Chronotype Genetic Variant in PER2 is Associated with Intrinsic Circadian Period in Humans.' *Sci Rep.* 2019; 9(1):5350.

21 Ashbrook L.H., Krystal A.D., Fu Y.H., et al. 'Genetics of the human circadian clock and sleep homeostat.' *Neuropsychopharmacology.* 2020; 45(1):45–54.

22 Patel S.R., Malhotra A., White D.P., et al. 'Association between reduced sleep and weight gain in women.' *American Journal of Epidemiology.* 2006; 164(10):947–54.

23 Cooper C.B., Neufeld E.V., Dolezal B.A., et al. 'Sleep deprivation and

obesity in adults: a brief narrative review.' *BMJ Open Sport & Exercise Medicine*. 2018;4(1).

24 Koren D., Dumin M., Gozal D. 'Role of sleep quality in the metabolic syndrome.' *Diabetes, Metabolic Syndrome and Obesity: Targets and Therapy*. 2016; 9:281.

25 Westerterp-Plantenga M.S. 'Sleep, circadian rhythm and body weight: parallel developments.' *Proc Nutr Soc*. 2016; 75(4):431–439.

26 Potter G.D., Skene D.J., Arendt J., et al. 'Circadian Rhythm and Sleep Disruption: Causes, Metabolic Consequences, and Countermeasures.' *Endocr Rev*. 2016; 37(6):584–608.

27 Peschke E., Peschke D. 'Evidence for a circadian rhythm of insulin release from perifused rat pancreatic islets.' *Diabetologia*. 1998; 41(9):1085–92.

28 Sadacca L.A., Lamia K.A., deLemos A.S., et al. 'An intrinsic circadian clock of the pancreas is required for normal insulin release and glucose homeostasis in mice.' *Diabetologia*. 2011; 54(1):120–4.

29 Rakshit K., Qian J., Ernst J., Matveyenko A.V. 'Circadian variation of the pancreatic islet transcriptome.' *Physiol Genomics*. 2016; 48(9):677–87.

30 Boden G., Ruiz J., Urbain J.L., et al. 'Evidence for a circadian rhythm of insulin secretion.' *Am J Physiol*. 1996; 271(2 Pt 1):E246–52.

31 Saad A., Dalla Man C., Nandy D.K., et al. 'Diurnal pattern to insulin secretion and insulin action in healthy individuals.' *Diabetes*. 2012; 61(11):2691–2700.

32 Rakshit K., Matveyenko A.V. 'Induction of Core Circadian Clock Transcription Factor Bmal1 Enhances β-Cell Function and Protects Against Obesity-Induced Glucose Intolerance.' *Diabetes*. 2021; 70(1):143–154.

33 Jakubowicz D., Wainstein J., Tsameret S., et al. 'Role of High Energy Breakfast "Big Breakfast Diet" in Clock Gene Regulation of Postprandial Hyperglycemia and Weight Loss in Type 2 Diabetes.' *Nutrients*. 2021; 13(5):1558.
Polonsky K.S., Given B.D., Van Cauter E. 'Twenty-four-hour profiles and pulsatile patterns of insulin secretion in normal and obese subjects.' *J Clin Invest*. 1988; 81(2):442–8.

36 Gale J.E., Cox H.I., Qian J., et al. 'Disruption of circadian rhythms accelerates development of diabetes through pancreatic beta-cell loss and dysfunction.' *J Biol Rhythms*. 2011; 26(5):423–33.

37 Shi S.Q., Ansari T.S., McGuinness O.P., et al. 'Circadian disruption leads to insulin resistance and obesity.' *Curr Biol*. 2013; 23(5):372–81.

38 Brainard J., Gobel M., Bartels K., et al. 'Circadian rhythms in anesthesia and critical care medicine: potential importance of circadian disruptions.' *Semin Cardiothorac Vasc Anesth*. 2015; 19(1):49–60.

39 Egi M., Bellomo R., Stachowski E., et al. 'Circadian rhythm of blood glucose values in critically ill patients.' *Crit Care Med*. 2007; 35(2):416–21.

40 Hung E.W., Aronson K.J., Leung M., et al. 'Shift work parameters and disruption of diurnal cortisol production in female hospital employees.' *Chronobiol Int*. 2016; 33(8):1045–55.

41 Ditzen B., Hoppmann C., Klumb P. 'Positive couple interactions and daily cortisol: on the stress-protecting role of intimacy.' *Psychosom Med*. 2008; 70(8):883–889.

42 Charlot A., Hutt F., Sabatier E., et al. 'Beneficial Effects of Early Time-Restricted Feeding on Metabolic Diseases: Importance of Aligning Food Habits with the Circadian Clock.' *Nutrients*. 2021; 13(5):1405.

43 Gill S., Panda S. 'A Smartphone App Reveals Erratic Diurnal Eating Patterns in Humans that Can Be Modulated for Health Benefits.' *Cell Metab*. 2015; 22(5):789–98.

44 Kolbe I., Brehm N., Oster H. 'Interplay of central and peripheral circadian clocks in energy metabolism regulation.' *J Neuroendocrinol*. 2019; 31(5):e12659.

45 Moon S., Kang J., Kim S.H., et al. 'Beneficial Effects of Time-Restricted Eating on Metabolic Diseases: A Systemic Review and Meta-Analysis.' *Nutrients*. 2020; 12(5):1267.

46 Adafer R., Messaadi W., Meddahi M., et al. 'Food Timing, Circadian Rhythm and Chrononutrition: A Systematic Review of Time-Restricted Eating's Effects on Human Health.' *Nutrients*. 2020; 12(12):3770.

47 Wilkinson M.J., Manoogian E.N.C., Zadourian A., et al. 'Ten-Hour Time-Restricted Eating Reduces Weight, Blood Pressure, and Atherogenic Lipids in Patients with Metabolic Syndrome.' *Cell Metab*. 2020; 31(1):92–104.e5.

48 Vollmers C., Gill S., DiTacchio L., et al. 'Time of feeding and the intrinsic circadian clock drive rhythms in hepatic gene expression.' *Proc Natl Acad Sci USA*. 2009; 106(50):21453–8.

49 Buettner D., Skemp S. 'Blue Zones: Lessons From the World's Longest Lived.' *Am J Lifestyle Med*. 2016; 10(5):318–321.

50 Willcox B.J., Willcox D.C., Todoriki H., et al. 'Caloric restriction, the traditional Okinawan diet, and healthy aging: the diet of the world's longest-lived people and its potential impact on morbidity and life span.' *Ann N Y Acad Sci*. 2007; 1114:434–455.

51 Chaix A., Manoogian E.N.C., Melkani G.C., et al. 'Time-Restricted Eating to Prevent and Manage Chronic Metabolic Diseases.' *Annu Rev Nutr*. 2019; 39:291–315.

52 Nagy A.D., Reddy A.B. 'Time dictates: emerging clinical analyses of the

impact of circadian rhythms on diagnosis, prognosis and treatment of disease.' *Clin Med* (Lond). 2015; 15 Suppl 6(0 6):s50–3.

53 St-Onge M.P., Ard J., Baskin M.L., et al: American Heart Association Obesity Committee of the Council on Lifestyle and Cardiometabolic Health; Council on Cardiovascular Disease in the Young; Council on Clinical Cardiology; and Stroke Council. 'Meal Timing and Frequency: Implications for Cardiovascular Disease Prevention: A Scientific Statement From the American Heart Association.' *Circulation*. 2017; 135(9):e96–e121.

54 Schuppelius B., Peters B., Ottawa A., et al. 'Time Restricted Eating: A Dietary Strategy to Prevent and Treat Metabolic Disturbances.' *Front Endocrinol* (Lausanne). 2021; 12:683140.

55 Pot G.K. 'Sleep and dietary habits in the urban environment: the role of chrono-nutrition.' *Proc Nutr Soc*. 2018; 77(3):189–198.

56 Gill S., Panda S. 'A Smartphone App Reveals Erratic Diurnal Eating Patterns in Humans that Can Be Modulated for Health Benefits.' *Cell Metab*. 2015; 22(5):789–98.

57 CHAPTER 15

1 Asbjørnsen R.A., Smedsrød M.L., Solberg Nes L., et al. 'Persuasive System Design Principles and Behavior Change Techniques to Stimulate Motivation and Adherence in Electronic Health Interventions to Support Weight Loss Maintenance: Scoping Review.' *J Med Internet Res*. 2019 Jun 21; 21(6).

2 Koliaki C., Spinos T., Spinou M., et al. 'Defining the Optimal Dietary Approach for Safe, Effective and Sustainable Weight Loss in Overweight and Obese Adults.' *Healthcare* (Basel). 2018 Jun 28; 6(3):73.

3 McLean N., Griffin S., Toney K., et al. 'Family involvement in weight control, weight maintenance and weight-loss interventions: a systematic review of randomised trials.' *Int J Obes Relat Metab Disord*. 2003 Sep; 27(9):987–1005.

4 Aronne L.J., Wadden T., Isoldi K.K., et al. 'When prevention fails: obesity treatment strategies.' *Am J Med*. 2009 Apr; 122(4 Suppl 1):S24–32.

CHAPTER 16

1 Goday A., Bellido D., Sajoux I., et al. 'Short-term safety, tolerability and efficacy of a very low-calorie-ketogenic diet interventional weight loss program versus hypocaloric diet in patients with type 2 diabetes mellitus.' *Nutr Diabetes*. 2016 Sep 19; 6(9).

2 Kuchkuntla A.R., Shah M., Velapati S., et al. 'Ketogenic Diet: an Endocrinologist Perspective.' *Curr Nutr Rep*. 2019 Dec; 8(4):402–410.

3 A reference paper on the subject of water intake, by the Institute of Medicine of the National Academies, is available at http://nap.edu/10925

4   Bostock E.C.S., Kirkby K.C., Taylor B.V., et al. 'Consumer Reports of "Keto Flu" Associated With the Ketogenic Diet.' *Front Nutr.* 2020 Mar 13; 7:20.

5   Harvey C.J.D.C., Schofield G.M., Zinn C., et al. 'Effects of differing levels of carbohydrate restriction on mood achievement of nutritional ketosis, and symptoms of carbohydrate withdrawal in healthy adults: A randomized clinical trial.' *Nutrition.* 2019; 67–68S:100005.

6   Paoli A., Bianco A., Damiani E., Bosco G. 'Ketogenic diet in neuromuscular and neurodegenerative diseases.' *Biomed Res Int.* 2014; 2014:474296.

7   Harvey C.J.D.C., Schofield G.M., Zinn C., et al. 'Effects of differing levels of carbohydrate restriction on mood achievement of nutritional ketosis, and symptoms of carbohydrate withdrawal in healthy adults: A randomized clinical trial.' *Nutrition.* 2019; 67–68S:100005.

8   Di Raimondo D., Buscemi S., Musiari G., et al. 'Ketogenic Diet, Physical Activity, and Hypertension-A Narrative Review.' *Nutrients.* 2021 Jul 27; 13(8):2567.

9   Elizabeth L., Machado P., Zinöcker M., et al. 'Ultra-Processed Foods and Health Outcomes: A Narrative Review.' *Nutrients.* 2020 Jun 30; 12(7):1955.

10 Swithers S.E. 'Artificial sweeteners are not the answer to childhood obesity.' *Appetite.* 2015 Oct; 93:85–90.

11 Malik V.S., Popkin B.M., Bray G.A., et al. 'Sugar-sweetened beverages and risk of metabolic syndrome and type 2 diabetes: a meta-analysis.' *Diabetes Care.* 2010 Nov; 33(11):2477–83.

12 Ibid.

13 Daher M.I., Matta J.M., Abdel Nour A.M. 'Non-nutritive sweeteners and type 2 diabetes: Should we ring the bell?' *Diabetes Res Clin Pract.* 2019 Sep; 155:107786.

14 Masood W., Annamaraju P., Uppaluri K.R. 'Ketogenic Diet.' [Updated 2021 Jun 11]. In: *StatPearls* [Internet]. Treasure Island (FL): StatPearls Publishing; 2021 Jan. Available from: https://www.ncbi.nlm.nih.gov/books/NBK499830

CHAPTER 18

1   Golbidi S., Daiber A., Korac B., et al. 'Health Benefits of Fasting and Caloric Restriction.' *Curr Diab Rep.* 2017 Oct 23; 17(12):123.

2   Hansen D., De Strijcker D., Calders P. 'Impact of Endurance Exercise Training in the Fasted State on Muscle Biochemistry and Metabolism in Healthy Subjects: Can These Effects be of Particular Clinical Benefit to Type 2 Diabetes Mellitus and Insulin-Resistant Patients?' *Sports Med.* 2017 Mar; 47(3):415–428.

3   Hoddy K.K., Marlatt K.L., Çetinkaya H., et al. 'Intermittent Fasting and

Metabolic Health: From Religious Fast to Time-Restricted Feeding.' *Obesity* (Silver Spring). 2020 Jul; 28 Suppl 1(Suppl 1):S29–S37.

4   Allaf M., Elghazaly H., Mohamed O.G., et al. 'Intermittent fasting for the prevention of cardiovascular disease.' *Cochrane Database of Systematic Reviews*. 2021 Jan 29; 1(1):CD013496.

5   Teong X.T., Liu K., Hutchison A.T., et al. 'Rationale and protocol for a randomized controlled trial comparing daily calorie restriction versus intermittent fasting to improve glycaemia in individuals at increased risk of developing type 2 diabetes.' *Obes Res Clin Pract*. 2020 Mar–Apr; 14(2):176–183.

6   Alhamdan B.A., Garcia-Alvarez A., et al. 'Alternate-day versus daily energy restriction diets: which is more effective for weight loss? A systematic review and meta-analysis.' *Obes Sci Pract*. 2016 Sep; 2(3):293–302.

FURTHER READING

The Telomere Effect, E. Blackburn and E. Epele (2017)

The Blue Zones: 9 Power Lesson For Living Longer From The People Who've Lived The Longest, D. Buettner (2012, second edition)

The Epigenetics Revolution, N. Carey (2012)

The Power of Habit, C. Duhigg (2012)

Run Stronger and Faster By Training Slower, M. Fitzgerald (2014)

The Obesity Code: Unlocking the Secrets of Weight Loss, J. Fung and T. Noakes (2016)

Fat Chance: The Hidden Truth About Sugar, Obesity and Disease, R. Lustig (2013)

Metabolical: The Truth About Processed Food and How it Poisons People and the Planet, R. Lustig (2021)

A Statin Free Life, A. Malhotra (2021)

Blueprint: How DNA Makes Us Who We Are, R. Plomin (2018)

'Unhappy Meals.' Michael Pollan. *The New York Times Magazine* (28 Jan 2007)

Why We Sleep: The New Science of Sleep and Dreams, M. Walker (2017)

Wooden: A Lifetime of Observations and Reflections On and Off the Court, J. Wooden and S. Jamison (1997)

ACKNOWLEDGEMENTS

You must be prepared to work always without applause.
Ernest Hemingway

We would like to thank all the scientists, doctors and researchers who share their knowledge to make the world a better place. Their dedication is truly inspirational. Without them this book could not exist and we are truly grateful. We also want to acknowledge patients who have shared their data and time so that mankind may benefit. We would like to thank the whisperers from all corners of the world who keep in touch. Your successes, enthusiasm and kind words touch our hearts.

Thank you.

All the mistakes in this book are our own. Apologies in advance.

INDEX

12-week reset plan: fasting 178–92
  food 162–70
  future 197–9
  meal plans 200–3
  weeks 1–4 171–7
  weeks 5–8 183–8
  weeks 9–12 189–96

absorption of nutrients 32–3
action plans 160, 169
addiction, to carbs and sugar 3
ageing 65
  autophagy 7–8, 126
agriculture 36–7
alcohol 27, 152, 190
alpha-linoleic acid (ALA) 55
amino acids 32, 63–4
anabolic hormones 102–3
antagonistic foods 33
antibiotics 71, 76
antidepressants 20, 73
artificial sweeteners 46–7, 165–6
asparagus: Sasfi's creamy garlic
    prawns 232–3
atherosclerosis 58
autophagy 7–8, 118, 126
avocados: prosciutto wrap 218–19

bacon: BLT wrap 218
  the full English breakfast 208
  grilled kippers with bacon and
    tomatoes 211–12

scrambled egg with bacon and
    mushrooms 206–7
bacteria *see* gut bugs
basal metabolic rate (BMR) 89, 167
beef: Bolognese sauce with cour-
    getti 234–5
  Christine's cottage pie 231
bioavailability 42–3, 44
blood glucose 43–6, 80
  carbohydrates and 40–1
  fasting and 122, 123–4, 125–6
  fizzy drink syndrome 105–7
  glycaemic index 43–4
  hormones and 98
  insulin and 103–6
  insulin resistance 99
  metabolic syndrome 18, 80
blood pressure 4, 18, 80, 82
BLT wrap 218
Blue Zones 5, 17, 131, 143
body clock 7, 130–44, 191–2
body fat 78–89
  diet myths 90–1
  as energy store 89
  fat adaptation 6, 111–19
  fat burning 114
  fat cells 88
  fat storage hormones 96–107
  gender differences 88
  types of 78–9
  visceral fat 78, 79–80, 81, 85
  see also metabolic syndrome

body mass index (BMI) 16, 80, 86
body shape index 87
Bolognese sauce with courgetti 234–5
bowel 29–34
brain 79
  body clock 131
  and cholesterol 4
  fasting and 122, 123, 124, 125
  and gut bugs 72–3
Brazil nuts: yoghurt breakfast bowl 205
bread 18, 19, 40
breakfast 7, 24, 117, 122, 188, 202–3, 204–12
broccoli, roast 246

cabbage: tuna and white cabbage salad 217
  white cabbage salad 225–6
calories 25–7, 91–4, 104, 105, 112, 166–7
cancer 5, 81
Caprese salad 224–5
Carbohydrate Insulin Model (CIM) 105
carbohydrates 24, 35–50
  bioavailability 42–3, 44
  calorie density 26
  carbohydrate revolutions 19
  classifying 40
  digestion 32
  and endurance sports 6
  and fat burning 114
  fat fuel inhibition 112–13
  fibre 41–2
  glycaemic index (GI) 43–4
  keto diet 166–7
  metabolic stress 48–9
  refined carbohydrates 2, 4, 19, 27, 35–6, 37, 39–40, 149, 198

  super-refined carbohydrates 19, 35–6, 37, 39–40, 149, 198
  what is a carbohydrate? 38
cardiovascular disease (CVD) 46, 82
catabolic hormones 102
cauliflower: cauliflower mashed 'potatoes' 241
  Christine's cottage pie 231
  shepherd's pie 229–30
celeriac mash 242
cells: autophagy 7–8, 118, 126
  circadian rhythm 130–1
  fasting and 122
  fat adaptation 117–18
cellulose 38, 41
charcuterie and cheese board 219–20
cheese: baked cod with chorizo topping 236–7
  charcuterie and cheese board 219–20
  cheese omelette 215
  classic Caprese salad 224–5
  frittata egg muffins 209
  Greek omelette 214–15
  Greek salad 223–4
chia seeds: noatmeal porridge 204
chicken: chicken tikka 235–6
  Greek marinated chicken 237–8
children, obesity 16, 87, 88, 105
chimichurri sauce 248–9
  salmon fillets with 233
cholesterol 4, 18, 52, 53, 57–9, 80, 198
chorizo, baked cod with 236–7
Christine's cottage pie 231
chrono-nutrition 142–4
chronotypes 136–7
circadian rhythm 76, 129–44
Clostridium difficile 71

coconut: crunchy nutty granola 210–11

coconut milk: noatmeal porridge 204

cod with chorizo topping 236–7

collagen 64

combination therapy 5

comfort eating 159–60

condiments 248–51

corn syrup 61, 88, 100, 149

cortisol 100–2, 137, 138, 139–40

cottage pie 231

courgettes: Bolognese sauce with courgetti 234–5

  courgetti 240

  frittata 216–17

Covid-19 pandemic 15

cravings 6, 173, 174–5, 176, 177

cucumber: Greek salad 223–4

  Turkish salad 222

death rates, obesity and 16, 80

deficiencies 199

depression 73

DEXA scans 85, 87

diabetes: hypoglycaemia 45

  insulin resistance 46

  metabolic syndrome and 82

diet whispering 21–2

diets: failure 1

  myths 90–5

  yo-yo dieting 65–6

digestion 32, 141

docosahexaenoic acid (DHA) 55

drinks 168

  alcohol 27, 152, 190

  artificial sweeteners 46–7, 165–6

  at bedtime 151

  fizzy drinks 3, 17, 26, 105–7, 165–6

  water 24, 127, 163–4, 179

  while fasting 127

EatSpan® 7, 116, 117, 121, 141, 142, 150

eggs: basic omelette 213–14

  frittata 216–17

  frittata egg muffins 209

  the full English breakfast 208

  green shakshuka 228–9

  poached egg, smoked salmon and spinach 205–6

  salad Niçoise 223

  scrambled egg with bacon and mushrooms 206–7

  traditional shakshuka 227–8

eicosapentaenoic acid (EPA) 55

Einstein, Albert 1

energy store, body fat as 89

enzymes 30, 32, 38, 114

epigenetics 14

exercise 4, 17, 76, 151

  and autophagy 8

  gyms 3, 92–4, 164

  metabolic syndrome and 82

  muscles 64

faecal transplants 71, 73

failure, dieting 159

farting 29, 42

fasting 8, 17, 76, 92, 120–8

  12-week reset plan 178–92

FastSpan® 7, 10, 116, 117, 121, 142, 143, 150

fat, body see body fat

fat adaptation 6, 111–19, 120, 149, 162

fat fuel inhibition 112–13

fats 24–5, 51–61

  calorie density 26

  cholesterol 4, 52, 53, 57–9

  digestion 32

  food list 168

  keto diet 166–7

  monosaturated fats 52, 53

myths and fats 51–2
and obesity 2
polyunsaturated fats 52, 53–7
saturated fats 2, 51, 52–3, 60–1
trans fats 52, 60
fennel, braised 243
fibre 33, 35, 38, 41–2, 71, 164, 199
fish 168
fizzy drinks 3, 17, 26, 105–7, 165–6
food 23–8, 168
12-week reset plan 162–70
and body clock 135
cravings 6, 173, 174–5, 176, 177
digestion 29
food diaries 150–1
high-quality versus low-quality 165
labels 47
macronutrients and micronutrients 24–5
meals 24
nutrient profiling 25–7
timing 131, 135, 140–2, 150, 154
whisperer plans 149, 154
frittata 216–17
frittata egg muffins 209
fructose 38–40, 42, 47–8, 61, 88, 149
fruit 168
fruit juice 42
the full English breakfast 208
fungal infections 81

galactose 38, 39
garlic mushrooms 244
genes 13, 72, 100, 113–14, 131
ghrelin 18, 91, 92, 98, 100, 106, 126, 141

glucagon 98, 103, 123, 125–6
glucose 18, 24, 38–9, 47
see also blood glucose
glycaemic index (GI) 43–4
glycaemic load (GL) 43–4
glycogen 38, 98, 114, 123, 124, 125
goals 155–61
granola, crunchy nutty 210–11
Greek marinated chicken 237–8
Greek omelette 214–15
Greek salad 223–4
green beans: haricots verts 247
salad Niçoise 223
green shakshuka 228–9
growth hormone 138, 140
gut 29–34
gut bugs 8, 21, 31–2, 69–77
and brain 72–3
circadian rhythm 130
and fibre 35, 42, 71
functions 72
helping 75–6
and immune system 72
keystone species 71, 74
metabolic syndrome and 82
and refined carbohydrates 36
and weight 73–5
gyms 3, 92–4, 164

ham: charcuterie and cheese board 219–20
prosciutto wrap 218–19
haricots verts 247
healthcare professionals 2, 20
heart disease 18, 46, 56–7, 58, 61, 82
hormones 6, 8, 21
blood glucose levels 45
and body fat 79, 80
and calorie restricting 91–2
circadian rhythm 138
diet myths 95
and fat adaptation 114

fat storage hormones 96–107
   functions 96–7
   ghrelin 18, 91, 92, 98, 100,
      106, 126, 141
   leptin 88, 100, 106, 141
hospitals 20
hunger 18, 100, 106, 122, 153
hypoglycaemia 45–6, 98

immune system 15, 30, 72
inflammation 53–5, 72
insulin 97–8
   and circadian rhythm 138, 139
   fasting and 122, 125, 126
   food and 103–6, 114
insulin resistance 14, 46, 98–9
   and body clock 136
   and circadian rhythm 139
   fasting and 126
   gut bugs and 74
   and lack of sleep 137
   metabolic syndrome 84–5
intermittent fasting 124

jet lag 135–6, 139
juice, fruit 42
junk food *see* processed foods

kale: green shakshuka 228–9
keto flu 162–3, 173, 174
ketogenic diet 116–18, 162, 166–7
ketone bodies 123, 124, 126, 162,
   174, 176
ketosis 173
Keys, Ancel 60–1
kippers with bacon and tomatoes
   211–12

labels, food 47
lamb: shepherd's pie 229–30
large intestine 30–1
late-night eating 142

leaky gut 30
leeks, buttered 239
leptin 88, 100, 106, 141
lettuce: BLT wrap 218
life expectancy 6, 17, 74
light, and body clock 7, 132–3,
   135
lipoproteins 57–9
liver: and cholesterol 4
   fat stores 78
   fructose and 40
   glycogen 114, 123, 124
low-fat foods 51–2, 61, 149, 168
lunch 117, 139, 150, 202–3,
   213–20
lysosomes 7–8

macronutrients 24–5, 26, 198
meal plans 200–3
meals, definition 24
mealtimes 7, 139, 141–2, 150
measurements 153
meat 56, 64, 168
Mediterranean diet 53, 116, 143
melanopsin 132–3
melatonin 137, 138
men, body fat 88
metabolic stress 48–9
metabolic syndrome 14, 18–19
   causes 84–5
   consequences of 81–3
   definition 80
   tests 85–8
metabolically obese normal weight
   (MONW) 14, 80
metabolism 1–2
   basal metabolic rate 89, 167
   and causes of obesity 2
   circadian rhythm 138–40
   insulin resistance and 14
   whisperer reset plan 15
microbiome *see* gut bugs

micronutrients 25, 26
minerals 25
mint yoghurt 251
mitochondria 117–18
monounsaturated fats 52, 53
mood changes 153
morbid obesity 86
motivation 155–6
muffins, frittata egg 209
multinationals 20–1
muscles 64–7, 78, 93, 113, 151–2
mushrooms: frittata egg muffins
    209
  the full English breakfast 208
  garlic mushrooms 244
  mushroom omelette 215
  scrambled egg with bacon and
    mushrooms 206–7

net carbs 38, 166, 167
noatmeal porridge 204
nutrient density 25–6
nutrional deficiencies 199
nuts 168
  crunchy nutty granola 210–11

obesity 13–19
  body mass index 86
  causes 2, 14
  in children 16
  circadian rhythm and 140–1
  costs of 15–16
  and death 16
  metabolic stress 48–9
oils 168
olives: Greek omelette 214–15
  Greek salad 223–4
omega-3 fatty acids 6, 53–7, 149
omega-6 fatty acids 53–7, 149,
    165
omelettes: basic omelette 213–14
  Greek omelette 214–15

onion raita 221–2

parsley: chimichurri 248–9
partners 153
peppers: traditional shakshuka
    227–8
plate portions 167
polyunsaturated fats 52, 53–7
porridge, noatmeal 204
prawns, Sasfi's creamy garlic 232–3
pregnancy 14, 181
probiotics 76
processed foods 2, 3, 19, 39–40,
    74, 165, 168, 169
prosciutto wrap 218–19
proteins 25, 63–8
  calorie density 26
  digestion 32
  food list 168
  functions 64
  keto diet 166–7
  protein shakes 152
  quantities 67
  supplements 67

raita, onion 221–2
raspberries: yoghurt breakfast bowl
    205
refined carbohydrates 2, 4, 19, 27,
    35–6, 37, 39–40, 149, 198
reflux 82
religion, and fasting 122–3
resistance training 151–2

safety, low-carb diet 164
salads 221–6
  classic Caprese salad 224–5
  Greek salad 223–4
  onion raita 221–2
  salad Niçoise 223
  tuna and white cabbage salad
    217

Turkish salad 222
  white cabbage salad 225–6
salmon fillets with chimichurri
    sauce 233
salt 82
sarcopenia 65
Sasfi's creamy garlic prawns 232–3
satiety hormone 67, 88, 100, 106,
    141, 181
saturated fats 2, 51, 52–3, 60–1
sauces 168
sausages: the full English breakfast
    208
scans, metabolic syndrome 85–6,
    87
screens, blue light 132–3
seeds 168
  crunchy nutty granola 210–11
serotonin 20, 73
shakshuka: green shakshuka
    228–9
  traditional shakshuka 227–8
shepherd's pie 229–30
shift work 136
sleep 20, 76, 81, 132–3, 136–8,
    140
sleep apnoea 81
small intestine 30, 31, 32–3
smoked salmon: poached egg,
    smoked salmon and spinach
    205–6
smoking 17, 21
snacks 7, 18, 24, 105, 140, 142,
    151, 159–60
snoring 81
social jet lag 135–6
societal change 5
spinach: frittata egg muffins 209
  poached egg, smoked salmon
    and spinach 205–6
  spinach omelette 215
starch 38

statins 4, 59
stomach 30, 32
stools 41, 42
stress, and cortisol 139–40
subcutaneous fat 78, 79
sucrose 39, 40
sugar 2, 21, 25–6, 38–9, 149, 169,
    174–5
super-refined carbohydrates 19,
    35–6, 37, 39–40, 149, 198
supermarkets 17
supper 24, 139, 202–3, 227–38
supplements 67, 127
support groups 153
sweeteners, artificial 46–7, 165–6
synergistic foods 33

teenagers, obesity 88, 105–6
telomeres 100
time 133–5
tinned foods 200–1
tomatoes: BLT wrap 218
  Bolognese sauce with courgetti
    234–5
  classic Caprese salad 224–5
  the full English breakfast 208
  Greek omelette 214–15
  Greek salad 223–4
  grilled kippers with bacon and
    tomatoes 211–12
  onion raita 221–2
  salad Niçoise 223
  scrambled egg with bacon and
    mushrooms 206–7
  tomato sauce 249–50
  traditional shakshuka 227–8
  Turkish salad 222
trans fats 52, 60
treat meals 154, 159, 180, 190,
    191–2, 201
triggers 159–60
triglycerides 18, 40, 51, 58, 80

tryptophan 20, 73
tuna: salad Niçoise 223
    tuna and white cabbage salad
        217
Turkish salad 222

vagus nerve 72–3
vegetables 168, 239–47
    roast vegetables 245
vegetarian diet 55
vinaigrette dressing 250–1
visceral fat 18–19, 78, 79–80, 81,
        85
vitamins 25, 79, 127

waist circumference 86, 175
waist-to-hip ratio 86–7, 175
water 24, 127, 163–4, 179
weight: diet myths 90–5
    and gut bugs 73–5
    insulin and 104
    insulin resistance and 14
    and mealtimes 139

weight loss journals 157–8,
        192
whisperer plans 147–9
whey protein 67
whisperer-loss plan 147–9, 165
whisperer-recover plan 147–8, 198
whisperer-stable-active plan 198
whisperer-stable plan 127, 147–8,
        164–5
whisperer-stable-regular plan 198
women, body fat 88
work, and body clock 136
World Health Organization (WHO)
        16, 60, 86–7
wraps 218–19

yo-yo dieting 65–6
yoghurt 61, 112
    mint yoghurt 251
    yoghurt breakfast bowl 205
Yudkin, John 60

zeitgebers, body clock 131–2